D1547379

Practical Guide to

Essential Oils

with References and Traditional Uses

©2016 by RM Barry Publications, LLC

Table of Contents

Chapter 1

The Best of Science and Nature

Plants have been used for thousands of years to help heal and calm. We can imagine early man making extracts from stems, leaves, barks and roots, and noting which reduced pain, which reduced swelling, which were calming and which were stimulating. By trial and error, remedies were discovered and recipes of cherished traditional treatments were passed on from generation to generation.

Ancient civilizations developed methods to extract plant essences. They gathered olives and pressed them into olive oil, and used olive oil for food, ointments and perfumed oils. In 2003 the remains of the world's oldest "perfume making factory" was found at Pyrgos, Cyprus. *The Age* reports that in 1850 BC a violent earthquake covered the site with earth. From the residues found at the amazingly well-preserved site, four perfumes were recreated. They "distilled them according to techniques described by Pliny the Elder (A.D. 23-79), by grinding the herbs, adding them to oil and water, and burying them in a long-necked jug over hot embers for twelve hours."[1] The methods and results are quite different from modern distilled oils that are produced today.

Research is beginning to explain some of the mystery behind the art and science of essential oil therapy. According to the University of Maryland Medical Center it is not entirely clear how aromatherapy or the use of essential oils work. Some researchers believe that when we inhale essential oils, molecules communicate with our brain and stimulate the parts of our brain "that serve as storehouses for emotions and memories."[2]

A 2013 study found that inhaling diffused rosemary essential oil improved memory. Significant amounts of 1,8-cineole, a compound found in rosemary oil, were found in blood tests of those who inhaled the rosemary oil. This suggests that memory was improved by absorption of compounds found in rosemary essential oil.[3]

Powerful Essences

It takes 600 pounds of rose flowers to produce 1 ounce (30 ml which is 2 tablespoons) of rose oil.[4]

It takes 16 pounds of peppermint leaf to produce 1 ounce of peppermint oil.[5]

Essential oils are so concentrated they are used by the counted-drop. Before we go further into the amazing world of essential oils, let's look at some basic recommendations:

Pay attention to the product safety label: Keep out of reach of children. Avoid contact with eyes.

Do not take by mouth. Even though an essential oil may be sourced from an edible plant, essential oils are very concentrated and should only be taken by mouth as directed by a healthcare provider.

The FDA does recognize some essential oils as GRAS (generally recognized as safe). GRAS-designated essential oils are used by the food industry in small amounts as food flavoring and are not intended to be ingested as health-benefiting remedies.

Pregnancy and Nursing. The use of essential oils when pregnant is generally not recommended, as essential oil compounds can cross the placental barrier and cross into breast milk. Consult a healthcare provider before using any essential oil when pregnant. The National Association for Holistic Aromatherapy explains that some essential oils appear to be safe for use when pregnant. They also warn that "It would be prudent to avoid the internal or undiluted application of essential oils throughout pregnancy." [6]

Children and Babies. Robert Tisserand and Rodney Young, authors of *Essential Oil Safety, A Guide for Health Care Professionals, 2nd Edition* explain that babies have thinner, more permeable skin than adults, and are more vulnerable to skin damage from products applied to their skin. Essential oils should be more diluted when used on children under the age of fifteen.[7]

Frail, Elderly, or those taking prescription medicines would be wise to heed the saying, "start low and go slow."[8]

Application of Essential Oils

Depending on the compounds found in an essential oil, it can be used aromatically or topically. Most essential oils should not be applied neat or directly to the skin without being diluted in carrier oil. It is suggested that a drop or two of lavender essential oil or tea tree oil can be used undiluted on a bite or a sting, or on a small area. Although not common, using any oil excessively for a long period of time can trigger a skin-sensitization reaction, which is an allergy-like inflammatory reaction.

Carrier Oils

Carrier oils are used to dilute essential oils and to carry the blend on the skin. As with all oils, carrier oils can become rancid or oxidized, so it is best to purchase them in small quantities and store them in a cool dark place. When preparing lution, first measure the correct amount of carrier oil in a glass container, and en add the suggested amount of essential oil drops. Both sweet almond oil and actionated coconut oil are good carrier oils, and are moisturizing.

Sweet Almond Oil is anti-inflammatory and believed to reduce scarring, reju- enate skin and is traditionally used to treat dry skin conditions.[9]

Fractionated Coconut Oil stays liquid and feels light on the skin. It is widely sed in cosmetics and aromatherapy.[10]

Dilutions for Use on Skin

Most essential oils need to be diluted with carrier oil before applying to the kin. The amount of dilution depends on the oil used, the age and health condition f the person using the oil, and the purpose of the use.

General Recommendations

Check individual oils for safety recommendations. According to Robert isserand and Rodney Young, 30 ml is estimated to be the maximum amount of a iluted blend that should be used in one day.[11]

How to Calculate a Dilution

To make your desired dilution, use the following chart as a guide. Add drops to arrier oil and shake or mix well. Use an accurate measuring device, not silverware.

Dilution Percentage	0.5%	1%	2%	3%	5%
EO for 2 tsp (10 ml) carrier oil	1 drop	3 drops	6 drops	9 drops	15 drops
EO for 1/2 oz (15 ml) carrier oil	2 drops	4 drops	9 drops	13 drops	22 drops
EO for 1 oz (30 ml) carrier oil	4 drops	9 drops	18 drops	27 drops	45 drops

NOTE: EO=Essential Oil. These values are approximate and have been rounded) whole drops. A drop is not a precise measure. Does not imply that all these ilutions are safe for all essential oils in all situations.[12]

Overexposure: It is possible to be overexposed to essential oils. Researchers ad a hundred spa workers sit in a room and breathe the vapors of bergamot oil r two hours. After the first hour they noted that the workers heart rate and blood ressure went down. After two hours researchers noted that blood pressure and eart rate had risen higher than at the beginning of the study.[13]

Bath: Usually 2 to 5 drops of essential oil, combined with a dispersing agent ich as a teaspoon of whole milk, vegetable oil, or even honey, are added to a full ath. Undiluted oils can float on top of the water and come in direct contact with skin. Some undiluted oils may be irritating.

Add oils to a full bath. If oils are added as the bath is filling, the agitation of the water can vaporize some of the essential oil.

Diffusing: Follow the instructions that came with the diffuser. To avoid over exposure run the diffuser for only 15 to 20 minutes.

Direct Inhalation: Add a few drops to a handkerchief, tissue or cotton ball and inhale the aroma of the oil. If you choose to inhale the aroma directly from the bottle, hold the bottle a few inches below your nose and take a quick sniff or two. Be careful not to ingest the oil through your nose as that can be toxic.

About Humidifiers: Not all humidifiers are made for use with essential oils. Adding oil to the water tank can damage the humidifier.

Steam Inhalation Congestion: The National Association for Holistic Aroma therapy recommends adding three to seven drops of essential oil and boiling water to a bowl. Make a tent with a towel over your head and bowl of water, close eyes and breathe the steam. (Use oils recommended for steam inhalation).[14]

Home Spray: Essential oils can be mixed with a small amount of water, well shaken and used as a quick spray. This will work for a short period of time.

A better spray can be made by mixing essential oils with grain alcohol or high proof vodka. Essential oils readily dissolve in alcohol and will keep longer. Do not use isopropyl alcohol. You can make up different mixtures, for example one to energize and stimulate, one to help calm and relax, and one to use as a room spray during cold and flu season. For each mixture you will need a small (4 ounce) glass spray bottle or plant mister. When making up a home spray, take into consideration the safety information of each essential oil. What you spray into the air will come into contact with people, surfaces, and potentially food and beverages that are in the room.

To make a home spray, combine:
- 2 ounces (4 tablespoons) distilled water
- 1 ounce (2 tablespoons) high proof vodka
- 20 to 30 drops of your favorite essential oil or a mix of oils
- Shake well before each use.[15]

How to Choose an Essential Oil

The label should state 100% essential oil.

The botanical name of the plant should be included along with the common name. Listing the botanical name is needed in order to determine exactly what compounds are contained in the oil. Different plant parts, extraction methods and even the country where the plant was grown can cause the oil to vary in composition. Therefore the country of origin, the parts of the plants used and the extraction method should be listed.

Essential Oil Chemistry

An individual essential oil may contain up to two hundred chemical constituents or naturally occurring compounds.[16] Compounds are what give individual oils their qualities. Aromatic compounds not only give plants their unique smell, but also help attract plant pollinators and deter damaging insects.

Understanding the naturally occurring chemistry of an essential oil gives clues about how to use the essential oil. For instance, are the chemical compounds anti-microbial? Are they known to soothe the skin? Do they repel or kill insects? Are they known to relax, stimulate, lower blood pressure or decongest a stuffy nose?

In a world where antibiotic resistance is becoming more and more common, scientists are investigating the properties of essential oils. In ancient times trial and error may have determined the medicinal use of plants. In the present day medicinal properties can be determined by chemically analyzing an essential oil. Today researchers can look at both the traditional use and the chemical composition of an essential oil and conduct studies that are, in some cases, providing scientific support for use of the oil.

References

http://www.theage.com.au/news/world/4000yearold-perfumes-found-on-aphrodites-fabled-island/2007/03/21/1174153159639.html

Source: Aromatherapy | University of Maryland Medical Center http://umm.edu/health/medical/altmed/treatment/aromatherapy#ixzz3ZaSVn8q8

British Psychological Society (BPS). "Rosemary aroma may help you remember to do things". Science-Daily. ScienceDaily, 9 April 2013. www.sciencedaily.com/releases/2013/04/130409091104.htm .

http://scienceline.org/2013/01/making-scents-the-aromatic-world-of-flowers/

http://www.dummies.com/how-to/content/understanding-essential-oils.html

https://www.naha.org/explore-aromatherapy/safety/#pregnancy

Tisserand, Robert; Young, Rodney. Essential Oil Safety: A Guide for Health Care Professionals. Elsevier Health Sciences UK 2nd Edition 2014, page 47

http://www.modernmedicine.com/content/polypharmacy-keeping-elderly-safe

The uses and properties of almond oil. Ahmad Z.
Complement Ther Clin Pract. 2010 Feb;16(1):10-2.
doi: 10.1016/j.ctcp.2009.06.015. Epub 2009 Jul 15.
PMID:20129403

https://www.organicfacts.net/health-benefits/oils/fractionated-coconut-oil.html

Tisserand, Robert and Rodney Young. Essential Oil Safety: A Guide for Health Care Professionals. 2nd Edition. Edinburgh: Churchill Livingston Elsevier Health Sciences. 2014. Print. Page 189

Tisserand, Robert and Rodney Young. Essential Oil Safety: A Guide for Health Care Professionals. 2nd Edition. Edinburgh: Churchill Livingston Elsevier Health Sciences. 2014. Print. Page 48

http://www.livescience.com/25174-essential-oils-heart-health.html

https://www.naha.org/explore-aromatherapy/about-aromatherapy/methods-of-application/

http://organicconnectmag.com/project/make-your-own-aromatherapy-room-spray/

Tisserand, Robert and Rodney Young. Essential Oil Safety: A Guide for Health Care Professionals. 2nd Edition. Edinburgh: Churchill Livingston Elsevier Health Sciences. 2014. Print. Page 21

Chapter 2

Bergamot
Citrus bergamia

Botanical Family:	Rutaceae (Citrus)	**Country of Origin**:	Italy
Parts Used:	Fruit	**Extraction Method**:	Cold Pressed

History and Traditional Use

Bergamot oil comes from the peel of a small citrus tree widely grown on the southern coast of Italy. The citrus-scented oil is used in perfumes and cosmetics.

The main constituents are limonene and linalyl acetate. Patricia Davis, author of *Aromatherapy An A-Z*, writes that bergamot oil is useful for depression and anxiety.[17]

Research

Antimicrobial: Vapors of tea tree oil, bergamot, lavender and eucalyptus inhibited both bacteria and fungi.[18]

Anxiety: Bergamot essential oil aromatherapy lowered preoperative anxiety.[19]

Anxiety and Depression: Topically applied blended lavender and bergamot essential oils reduced heart rate and blood pressure. This blend may be used for treating depression and anxiety.[20]

Blood Pressure–Stress Management: For ten minutes fifty-four school teachers breathed a spray mist of bergamot essential oil. Results demonstrated significant decreases in blood pressure and heart rate after application.[21]

Blood Pressure–Stress: Researchers found that persons with essential hypertension who once a day inhaled a combination of lavender, ylang-ylang and bergamot essential oils reduced psychological stress as well as blood pressure.[22]

Dermatophytosis–Athlete's Foot, Ringworm: In a laboratory-conducted study bergamot oil was shown to be a potent antifungal agent against several species of dermatophytes.[23]

Hospice Care: Aromatherapy hand massage was beneficial for reducing pain and depression in hospice patients with terminal cancer. Each hand was massaged for five minutes with a blend of bergamot, lavender and frankincense essential oils. [24]

Safety Tips

* Do not take bergamot oil by mouth.
* Always use diluted.
* Avoid sun or tanning bed exposure for twelve hours after using bergamot essential oil on the skin. Bergamot oil can intensify the effects of UV light.
* Tisserand and Young recommend no more than 30ml (6 teaspoons) of a 0.4% dilution be used on the skin per day. They also suggest that old or oxidized oils be avoided. Bergamot oil should be kept in a refrigerator, stored in a dark airtight container.[25]

How To Use

To use on skin: In a glass container combine carrier oil with the amount of drops needed for your desired dilution.

To make a 0.4% dilution add 4 drops to 30ml (6 teaspoons) carrier oil or 2 drops to 15ml (3 teaspoons) carrier oil.

Diffusion: Follow the instructions that came with the diffuser. To avoid over-exposure run the diffuser for only 15 to 20 minutes.

Direct Inhalation: Add a few drops to a handkerchief, tissue or cotton ball and inhale the aroma of the oil. If you choose to inhale the aroma directly from the bottle, hold the bottle a few inches below your nose and take a quick sniff or two. Be careful not to ingest the oil through your nose as that can be toxic.

References

7. Davis, Patricia, and Sarah Budd. *Aromatherapy an A-Z*. London: Vermillion, 2005. Print. Page 55
8. Vapour phase: a potential future use for essential oils as antimicrobials?
   Laird K, Phillips C.
   Lett Appl Microbiol. 2012 Mar;54(3):169-74.
   doi: 10.1111/j.1472-765X.2011.03190.x. Epub 2012 Jan 6.
   PMID:22133088
9. The anxiolytic effect of aromatherapy on patients awaiting ambulatory surgery: a randomized controlled trial.
   Ni CH, Hou WH, Kao CC, Chang ML, Yu LF, Wu CC, Chen C.
   Evid Based Complement Alternat Med. 2013;2013:927419. doi: 10.1155/2013/927419. Epub 2013 Dec 17.
   PMID:24454517
10. Aroma-therapeutic effects of massage blended essential oils on humans
    Hongratanaworakit T.
    Nat Prod Commun. 2011 Aug;6(8):1199-204.
    PMID: 21922934
. Aromatherapy benefits autonomic nervous system regulation for elementary school faculty in taiwan.
    Chang KM, Shen CW.
    Evid Based Complement Alternat Med. 2011;2011:946537. doi: 10.1155/2011/946537. Epub 2011 Apr 10.
    PMID:21584196

22. [The effects of the inhalation method using essential oils on blood pressure and stress responses of clients with essential hypertension].
Hwang JH.
Taehan Kanho Hakhoe Chi. 2006 Dec;36(7):1123-34. Korean.
PMID:17211115

23. In vitro activity of Citrus bergamia (bergamot) oil against clinical isolates of dermatophytes.
Sanguinetti M, Posteraro B, Romano L, Battaglia F, Lopizzo T, De Carolis E, Fadda G.
J Antimicrob Chemother. 2007 Feb;59(2):305-8. Epub 2006 Nov 20.
PMID:17118937

24. [Effects of aroma hand massage on pain, state anxiety and depression in hospice patients with terminal cancer].
Chang SY.
Taehan Kanho Hakhoe Chi. 2008 Aug;38(4):493-502. Korean.
PMID:18753801

25. Tisserand, Robert and Rodney Young. *Essential Oil Safety: A Guide for Health Care Professionals.* 2nd Edition. Edinburgh: Churchill Livingston Elsevier Health Sciences. 2014. Print. Page 211

Chapter 3

Cedarwood
Juniperus virginiana

** btanical Family**: Cupressaceae (Eastern Red Cedar)   **Country of Origin**:   United States

rts Used: Bark   **Extraction Method**:   Steam Distillation

History and Traditional Uses

Cedarwood essential oil is not the same as atlas cedarwood essential oil (*Cedrus atlantica*). Cedarwood essential oil is extracted from *Juniperus virginiana*, commonly known as eastern red cedar tree.

The insect-repelling wood is commonly used in cedar drawers and pencils.[26]

It was believed that smoke from juniper trees prevented leprosy and plaque. In World War II, French nurses fumigated hospital rooms by burning juniper. Juniper used as an antiseptic.[27]

Research

Anti-inflammatory–Wound Healing: In traditional medicine junipers are used as an antiseptic, an antifungal and for wound healing. Cedarwood essential oil was found to have high anti-inflammatory activity.[28]

Hair Growth–Alopecia Areata: In this study one group massaged thyme, rosemary, lavender and cedarwood essential oils mixed with carrier oil on their scalp. The other group used only carrier oil. 43% of the patients massaging the essential oils on their scalp showed improvement versus 15% improvement in the carrier oil group.[29]

Insect Repellant–Ants: Cedarwood essential oil repels ants including red imported fire ants.[30]

Mood–Calming: This study found inhaling cedrol (extracted from cedarwood oil) decreased heart rate, blood pressure and respiratory rates.[31]

Safety Tips
* Do not take by mouth
* Do not use if pregnant or nursing.

How To Use
To use on skin: To make your desired dilution add drops to 30 ml carrier o and shake or mix well. Use a glass container and an accurate measuring devic not silverware.

30 ml is the equivalent of 1 ounce or 2 tablespoons or 6 teaspoons

Elderly, Frail, Sensitive Skin	3 to 9 drops	0.5% to 1% dilution
Healthy Adults	9 to 18 drops	1% to 2% dilution
Short term on area of concern	18 to 27 drops	2% to 3% dilution

For more information on dilution please see first chapter.

Bath: Add a few diluted drops to a bath

Diffusion: Follow the instructions that came with the diffuser. To avoid ove exposure run the diffuser for only 15 to 20 minutes.

Direct Inhalation: Add a few drops to a handkerchief, tissue or cotton ba and inhale the aroma of the oil. If you choose to inhale the aroma directly fro the bottle, hold the bottle a few inches below your nose and take a quick sniff o two. Be careful not to ingest the oil through your nose as that can be toxic.

Insect repellent: For immediate use make a spray with water and a few dro of cedarwood and, if desired, other insect-repelling essential oils such as lemo grass, peppermint, clove, patchouli or ylang ylang.

References

26. "Juniper." New World Encyclopedia, . 26 May 2014, 20:13 UTC. 18 May 2015, 01:51 <http://www. newworldencyclopedia.org/p/index.php?title=Juniper&oldid=981807>.

27. Castleman, Michael. The Healing Herbs, The Ultimate Guide to the Curative Power of Natures Medicines. Emmaus: Rodale Press, 1991. Print Page 225

28. Topical wound-healing effects and phytochemical composition of heartwood essential oils ofJuniper virginiana L., Juniperus occidentalis Hook., and Juniperus ashei J. Buchholz.
Tumen I, Süntar I, Eller FJ, Keleş H, Akkol EK.
J Med Food. 2013 Jan;16(1):48-55. doi: 10.1089/jmf.2012.2472.
PMID:23297713

29. Randomized trial of aromatherapy. Successful treatment for alopecia areata.
Hay IC, Jamieson M, Ormerod AD.
Arch Dermatol. 1998 Nov;134(11):1349-52.
PMID:9828867

30. Bioactivity of cedarwood oil and cedrol against arthropod pests.
Eller FJ, Vander Meer RK, Behle RW, Flor-Weiler LB, Palmquist DE.
Environ Entomol. 2014 Jun;43(3):762-6. doi: 10.1603/EN13270. Epub 2014 Mar 31.
PMID:24690252

31. Autonomic responses during inhalation of natural fragrance of Cedrol in humans.
Dayawansa S, Umeno K, Takakura H, Hori E, Tabuchi E, Nagashima Y, Oosu H, Yada Y, Suzuki T, Ono T, Nishijo H.
Auton Neurosci. 2003 Oct 31;108(1-2):79-86.
PMID:14614964#

Chapter 4

Cinnamon Bark

Cinnamomum verum

Botanical Family: Lauraceae (Ceylon Cinnamon)   **Country of Origin**: Sri Lanka

Parts Used: Bark   **Extraction Method**: Steam Distillation

History and Traditional Use

Cinnamon spice, the ground powder made from cinnamon bark, has bee[n] used since ancient times as a treatment for fever, diarrhea, and menstrual problem[s]. By the nineteenth century some American physicians were prescribing cinnamo[n] spice for stomach cramps, flatulence, nausea, vomiting, diarrhea and uterin[e] problems.[32]

Cinnamomum verum is "true cinnamon" or Ceylon cinnamon. The majo[r] component of cinnamon bark oil is cinnamaldehyde. It is commonly used as [a] commercial food flavoring.[33]

Research

Antibacterial: A study showed that Gram-positive and Gram-negative isolate[s] belonging to Staphylococcus, Enterococcus, Enterobacter and Acinetobacter wer[e] inhibited by cinnamon bark oil, and that cinnamon bark oil has strong antibacteri[al] properties. It is recommended for use as an antibacterial compound in hospit[al] disinfectants.[34]

Antibacterial–Hospital Acquired Infections: This study looked at th[e] activity of cinnamon, lavender and geranium essential oils against Acinetobacte[r] species, a principle bacteria found in hard-to-treat hospital acquired infections. A[ll] three oils were effective. Cinnamon bark oil was the most effective.[35]

Antibacterial–Respiratory Infections: Fourteen essential oils were teste[d] against bacteria that cause respiratory infections. Thyme, cinnamon bark, lem[on]ongrass, perilla, and peppermint oils were found effective and chosen for furthe[r] evaluation.[36]

Antifungal–Candida albicans: Oregano, winter savory, peppermin[t]

cinnamon bark and lemongrass were found to be most effective against Candida albicans.[37]

Antimicrobial, Anti-tumor: In a laboratory-conducted study, cinnamon bark essential oil was found to have strong antimicrobial activity against twenty-one types of bacteria and four Candida species. The oil also showed anti-tumor activity.[38]

Safety Tips

- Do not take cinnamon bark oil by mouth.
- Do not use if pregnant or nursing.
- Do not use on children.
- This oil requires careful dilution.
- Do not use on diseased, damaged or broken skin.

Experts and authors have different opinions when it comes to using cinnamon bark essential oil. It is not recommended for use in massage or bath because cinnamon bark oil can be very irritating. Still, some experts praise the virtues of cinnamon bark oil.

Cinnamon bark oil is a known skin sensitizer. If used too frequently on skin without enough dilution, or on skin that is damaged, cinnamon bark oil can trigger the immune system to identify the oil as harmful and cause an allergy-like inflammatory reaction. This reaction is more common in persons who tend to have allergies. Tisserand and Young recommend no more than 30ml (6 teaspoons) of a 0.05% dilution be used on the skin per day.[39]

Cinnamon bark oil has strong antibacterial properties. With proper dilution and caution it may be a useful tool in our arsenal of home remedies.

How To Use

To use on skin: To make a 0.05% dilution add 1 drop to 60 ml carrier oil. This a much diluted solution. 60 ml is 2 ounces or 4 tablespoons or 12 teaspoons.

Diffusing: It is likewise important to be careful when diffusing cinnamon bark oil. Cinnamon bark oil can be drying and irritating to the protective mucous membranes found in our eyes, nose and mouth.[40] To reduce airborne-microbes, diffuse cinnamon bark oil for a few minutes in a well-ventilated room. Note the safety concern for young children and if pregnant.

Laundry and Cleaning: To disinfect laundry, add a couple of drops to the washing machine.

References

1. Castleman, Michael. *The Healing Herbs, The Ultimate Guide to the Curative Power of Natures Medicines*. Emmaus: Rodale Press, 1991. Print Page 116

2. http://www.fao.org/docrep/v5350e/v5350e04.htm

34. [The antibacterial activity of cinnamon oil on the selected gram-positive and gram-negative bacteria].
Urbaniak A, Głowacka A, Kowalczyk E, Lysakowska M, Sienkiewicz M.
Med Dosw Mikrobiol. 2014;66(2):131-41. Polish.
PMID:25369660

35. The biological activities of cinnamon, geranium and lavender essential oils.
Sienkiewicz M, Głowacka A, Kowalczyk E, Wiktorowska-Owczarek A, Jóźwiak-Bębenista M, Łysakowska M.
Molecules. 2014 Dec 12;19(12):20929-40. doi: 10.3390/molecules191220929.
PMID:25514231

36. Screening of the antibacterial effects of a variety of essential oils on respiratory tract pathogens, using a modified dilution assay method.
Inouye S, Yamaguchi H, Takizawa T.
J Infect Chemother. 2001 Dec;7(4):251-4.
PMID:11810593

37. The inhibition of Candida albicans by selected essential oils and their major components.
Tampieri MP, Galuppi R, Macchioni F, Carelle MS, Falcioni L, Cioni PL, Morelli I.
Mycopathologia. 2005 Apr;159(3):339-45.
PMID:15883716

38. Composition, antimicrobial activity and in vitro cytotoxicity of essential oil from Cinnamomum zeylanicum Blume (Lauraceae).
Unlu M, Ergene E, Unlu GV, Zeytinoglu HS, Vural N. Food Chem Toxicol. 2010 Nov;48(11):3274-80. doi: 10.1016/j.fct.2010.09.001. Epub 2010 Sep 7.
PMID:20828600

39. Tisserand, Robert and Rodney Young. *Essential Oil Safety: A Guide for Health Care Professionals.* 2nd Edition. Edinburgh: Churchill Livingston Elsevier Health Sciences. 2014. Print. Page 248

40. https://www.naha.org/explore-aromatherapy/safety/#dermal

Chapter 5

Clove
Eugenia caryophyllata

Botanical Family:	Myrtaceae	**Country of Origin**:	Indonesia
Parts Used:	Leaf	**Extraction Method**:	Steam Distillation

History and Traditional Use

The use of clove as spice and medicine goes back to ancient times. Wars and explorations were launched in pursuit of spices. Cinnamon, nutmeg and clove are spices grown in tropical parts of the world. Clove spice has been used as a digestive aid and mosquito and moth repellent. Clove has antibacterial, anti-inflammatory, antiviral, antifungal and antiseptic properties. Some dentists use clove oil as a natural oral anesthetic. Eugenol is the principal constituents found in clove oil.[41]

Research

Anesthetic−Dental: A study found that clove gel and benzocaine worked similarly as a topical anesthetic before needle insertion.[42]

Antibacterial: In this study cinnamon, clove, geranium, lemon, lime, orange and rosemary oils were effective at fighting some bacteria. Cinnamon oil worked really well even at low doses. Cinnamon, clove and lime essential oils worked against gram-positive and gram-negative bacteria.[43]

Antimicrobial: Black pepper, clove, geranium, nutmeg, oregano, and thyme essential oils were examined for antibacterial activity against twenty-five different kinds of bacteria. The oils were effective against all the tested organisms. This included bacteria that affect plants and animals and cause food poisoning and food spoilage.[44]

Antiseptic: Clove essential oil was found effective as an antiseptic in oral infections and a potential topical antimicrobial.[45]

Insect Repellent−Paper Wasps and Yellow Jackets: A blend of clove, geranium and lemongrass oils, and also a blend of clove, geranium, lemongrass and rosemary oils totally blocked the attraction of wasps, yellow jackets and hornets.[46]

Menstrual Cramps: Massaging the abdomen with cinnamon, clove, rose, and lavender in a base of almond oil for seven days before menstruation alleviated menstrual pain and reduced the amount of menstrual bleeding.[47]

Scabies: Clove oil was highly toxic against scabies mites showing promise for use in a topical treatment for scabies.[48]

Tooth Decay and Periodontal Disease: Clove oil and eugenol are effective natural antibacterial agents against the bacteria that cause tooth decay and periodontal disease.[49]

Safety Tips

- Do not ingest.
- Do not use if pregnant or nursing.
- Use caution on sensitive skin, or on damaged broken skin.
- Not for use on children under the age of two.
- Clove essential oil should always be used diluted. Tisserand and Young recommend no more than 30ml (6 teaspoons) of a 0.6% dilution be used on the skin per day.[50]

How To Use

To use on skin: In a glass container combine carrier oil with the amount of drops needed for your desired dilution.

To make a 0.6% dilution add 5 drops to 30ml (6 teaspoons) carrier oil.

Insect Repellent: For immediate use make a spray with water and a few drops of clove oil and, if desired, other insect-repelling essential oils such as geranium lemongrass or rosemary.

Toothache: Clove essential oil is used to temporarily treat toothache. If used it should be carefully applied, just a diluted drop on a cotton swab until you can get to the dentist. It can cause burning and damage to lips and mouth. Taken in excess, it is toxic.[51]

References

41. http://www.indepthinfo.com/cloves/health.shtml
42. The effect of clove and benzocaine versus placebo as topical anesthetics.
    Alqareer A, Alyahya A, Andersson L.
    J Dent. 2006 Nov;34(10):747-50. Epub 2006 Mar 13.
    PMID:16530911
43. In vitro antibacterial activity of some plant essential oils.
    Prabuseenivasan S, Jayakumar M, Ignacimuthu S.
    BMC Complement Altern Med. 2006 Nov 30;6:39.
44. Antimicrobial agents from plants: antibacterial activity of plant volatile oils.
    Dorman HJ, Deans SG.
    J Appl Microbiol. 2000 Feb;88(2):308-16.
    PMID:10736000

45. Microbicide activity of clove essential oil (Eugenia caryophyllata).
    Nuñez L, Aquino MD.
    Braz J Microbiol. 2012 Oct;43(4):1255-60. doi: 10.1590/S1517-83822012000400003. Epub 2012 Jun 1.
    PMID:24031950

46. Essential oils and their compositions as spatial repellents for pestiferous social wasps.
    Zhang QH, Schneidmiller RG, Hoover DR.
    Pest Manag Sci. 2013 Apr;69(4):542-52. doi: 10.1002/ps.3411. Epub 2012 Oct 19.
    PMID: 23081867

47. The effect of aromatherapy abdominal massage on alleviating menstrual pain in nursing students: a prospective randomized cross-over study.
    Marzouk TM, El-Nemer AM, Baraka HN.
    Evid Based Complement Alternat Med. 2013;2013:742421. doi: 10.1155/2013/742421. Epub 2013 Apr 11.
    PMID:23662151

48. Acaricidal activity of eugenol based compounds against scabies mites.
    Pasay C, Mounsey K, Stevenson G, Davis R, Arlian L, Morgan M, Vyszenski-Moher D, Andrews K, McCarthy J.
    PLoS One. 2010 Aug 11;5(8):e12079. doi: 10.1371/journal.pone.0012079.
    PMID:20711455

49. Synergistic effect between clove oil and its major compounds and antibiotics against oral bacteria.
    Moon SE, Kim HY, Cha JD.
    Arch Oral Biol. 2011 Sep;56(9):907-16. doi: 10.1016/j.archoralbio.2011.02.005. Epub 2011 Mar 12.
    PMID:21397894

50. Tisserand, Robert and Rodney Young. *Essential Oil Safety: A Guide for Health Care Professionals.* 2nd Edition. Edinburgh: Churchill Livingston Elsevier Health Sciences. 2014. Print. Page 256

51. http://well.blogs.nytimes.com/2011/02/17/remedies-clove-oil-for-tooth-pain/?_r=0

Chapter 6

Eucalyptus
Eucalyptus globulus

Botanical Family:	Myrtaceae (Blue Gum Tree)	**Country of Origin**:	China
Parts Used:	Leaf, Twig	**Extraction Method**:	Steam Distillation

History and Traditional Use

Eucalyptus trees are fast growing trees and are among the tallest trees in the world. They are native to Australia. In the 1940s and '50s the trees were exported to other parts of the world as a reliable source of wood. Today most eucalyptus oils are produced in China.

The main component in eucalyptus is 1,8-cineole (eucalyptol). 1,8-cineole anti-inflammatory, analgesic (provides pain relief) and aromatic.

Eucalyptus oil is used as a decongestant for treating sinus infection and bronchitis. It is used as an expectorant and to prevent an asthma attack. It has antibacterial, antiviral and antiseptic qualities. It is also used topically as a mild pain reliever and to repel insects.[52]

Research

Analgesic, Anti-inflammatory: This study found that eucalyptus oil helped relieve pain and reduce inflammation.[53]

Antimicrobial: Vapors of tea tree oil, bergamot, lavender and eucalyptus inhibited both bacteria and fungi.[54]

Antimicrobial, Asthma, Bronchitis, COPD: 1,8-cineole and eucalyptus oil displayed antimicrobial effects against many bacteria, including Mycobacterium tuberculosis and methicillin-resistant Staphylococcus aureus (MRSA), viruses, and fungi (including Candida). Eucalyptus also displayed properties that are immune stimulating, anti-inflammatory, analgesic, spasmolytic (relieve or prevent spasm) and antioxidant. Inhaling eucalyptus oil vapors was found beneficial for respiratory problems.[55]

Arthritis, Pain, Depression: Using a blend of lavender, marjoram, eucalyptus rosemary, and peppermint oils diluted in carrier oil significantly lowered pain and depression.[56]

Asthma, COPD: Clinical evidence shows eucalyptol (main component in eucalyptus oil) is beneficial for use as a long-term therapy for preventing COPD "flare-ups" and for better asthma control.[57]

Headache: A blend of peppermint oil, eucalyptus oil and ethanol (alcohol) applied to the forehead and temple significantly reduced headache pain.[58]

Insect Repellent: Essential oils have been investigated for use as natural insect and arthropod repellents. (Ants, bed bugs, fleas, house flies, ticks and mosquitoes are arthropods.) Monoterpenes and sesquiterpenes appear to be insect-repelling compounds. Lemongrass, basil and eucalyptus essential oils contain compounds that are most noted as effective insect repellents.[59]

Insecticide—House fly: This study found eucalyptus oil has potential as an environmentally friendly house fly insecticide.[60]

Safety Tips

- Do not take eucalyptus oil by mouth. It is toxic if taken by mouth.
- Do not put eucalyptus oil on or close to the face of a child under the age of ten.[61]
- Using eucalyptus oil may be contraindicated if you are using topical 5-fluoro-uracil (a topical cancer treatment).[62]

How To Use

To use on skin: To make your desired dilution add drops to 30 ml carrier oil and shake or mix well. Use a glass container and an accurate measuring device, not silverware.

30 ml is the equivalent of 1 ounce or 2 tablespoons or 6 teaspoons

Elderly, Frail, Sensitive Skin	3 to 9 drops	0.5% to 1% dilution
Healthy Adults	9 to 18 drops	1% to 2% dilution
Short term on area of concern	18 to 27 drops	2% to 3% dilution

For more information on dilution please see first chapter.

Diffusion: Follow the instructions that came with the diffuser. To avoid over-exposure run the diffuser for only 15 to 20 minutes. Note the safety concern for children.

Direct Inhalation: Add a few drops to a handkerchief, tissue or cotton ball and inhale the aroma of the oil. If you choose to inhale the aroma directly from the bottle, hold the bottle a few inches below your nose and take a quick sniff or two. Be careful not to ingest the oil through your nose as that can be toxic.

Insect repellent: For immediate use, make a spray with water and a few drops eucalyptus oil and if desired other insect-repelling essential oils such as peppe mint, cedarwood, patchouli, geranium, lavender, rosemary or ylang ylang.

For steam inhalation add 5 to 7 drops of oil to 2 cups boiling water. Plac towel over head, close eyes and inhale steam.

Laundry: Add a few drops to laundry.

To fight a cold and get ready for bed: Add 1 cup Epsom Salts to a war bath.[63] Combine 3 drops tea tree oil, 3 drops eucalyptus oil and 3 dro lavender oil in 30ml carrier oil. (6 teaspoons) Massage on arms and legs. Relax a warm bath.

References

52.   http://oilhealthbenefits.com/eucalyptus-oil/

53.   Analgesic and anti-inflammatory effects of essential oils of Eucalyptus.
      Silva J, Abebe W, Sousa SM, Duarte VG, Machado MI, Matos FJ.
      J Ethnopharmacol. 2003 Dec;89(2-3):277-83.
      PMID:14611892

54.   Vapour phase: a potential future use for essential oils as antimicrobials?
      Laird K, Phillips C.
      Lett Appl Microbiol. 2012 Mar;54(3):169-74. doi: 10.1111/j.1472-765X.2011.03190.x. Epub 2012 Jan 6.
      PMID:22133088

55.   Immune-modifying and antimicrobial effects of Eucalyptus oil and simple inhalation devices.
      Sadlon AE, Lamson DW.
      Altern Med Rev. 2010 Apr;15(1):33-47. Review.
      PMID:20359267

56.   [The effects of aromatherapy on pain, depression, and life satisfaction of arthritis patients].
      Kim MJ, Nam ES, Paik SI.
      Taehan Kanho Hakhoe Chi. 2005 Feb;35(1):186-94. Korean.
      PMID: 15778570

57.   Anti-inflammatory properties of the monoterpene 1.8-cineole: current evidence for co-medication in inflammatory airway diseases.
      Juergens UR.
      Drug Res (Stuttg). 2014 Dec;64(12):638-46. doi: 10.1055/s-0034-1372609. Epub 2014 May 15.

58.   Effect of peppermint and eucalyptus oil preparations on neurophysiological and experimental algesi-metric headache parameters.
      Göbel H, Schmidt G, Soyka D.
      Cephalalgia. 1994 Jun;14(3):228-34; discussion 182.
      PMID:7954745

59.   Repellent activity of essential oils: a review.
      Nerio LS, Olivero-Verbel J, Stashenko E.
      Bioresour Technol. 2010 Jan;101(1):372-8. doi: 10.1016/j.biortech.2009.07.048. Epub 2009 Sep 2.
      Review.
      PMID: 19729299

60.   Compositional analysis and insecticidal activity of Eucalyptus globulus (family: Myrtaceae)essential oil against housefly (Musca domestica).
      Kumar P, Mishra S, Malik A, Satya S.
      Acta Trop. 2012 May;122(2):212-8. doi: 10.1016/j.actatropica.2012.01.015. Epub 2012 Feb 2.
      PMID:22326717

61. Tisserand, Robert and Rodney Young. Essential Oil Safety: A Guide for Health Care Professionals. 2nd Edition. Edinburgh: Churchill Livingston Elsevier Health Sciences. 2014. Print. Page 273

62. Eucalyptus | University of Maryland Medical Center http://umm.edu/health/medical/altmed/herb/eucalyptus#ixzz3aXUk9fOd

63. http://www.epsomsaltcouncil.org/news/articles/doctors_say_treat_colds_flu_with_epsom_salt.php

Chapter 7

Frankincense
Boswellia Carteri

Botanical Family:	Burseraceae	**Country of Origin**:	Somalia
Parts Used:	Gum	**Extraction Method**:	Steam Distillation

History and Traditional Uses

Frankincense has been treasured since ancient times for use in worship an[ ] medicine. The aromatic gum-resin comes from trees grown in Somalia, Yemen an[ ] Oman. The fragrant resin is harvested from milk-like liquid that oozes from cuts o[ ] the trunks of the trees. The liquid dries into the resin that is frankincense.[64]

Patricia Davis author of *Aromatherapy An A-Z* writes that frankincense essenti[ ] oil massage is useful for asthma relief because it is calming. It helps a person tak[ ] deeper breaths and slows breathing.[65]

Research

Antifungal: An investigation of several frankincense essential oils found tha[ ] Boswellia carteri (Somalia) had the best activity against fungal strains.[66]

Hospice Care: Aromatherapy hand massage was beneficial for treating pai[ ] and depression in hospice patients. Each hand was massaged for five minutes wit[ ] a blended mixture of bergamot, lavender and frankincense diluted with swee[ ] almond carrier oil.[67]

Safety Tips

- Do not take frankincense oil by mouth.
- Do not use rancid or oxidized oil.
- Tisserand and Young note that skin sensitization (allergy-like reaction) is possibl[ ] if oil is oxidized. Keep oil in a dark, airtight container in a refrigerator.[68]

How To Use

To use on skin: To make your desired dilution add drops to 30 ml carrier oil and shake or mix well. Use a glass container and an accurate measuring device, not silverware.

30 ml is the equivalent of 1 ounce or 2 tablespoons or 6 teaspoons

Elderly, Frail, Sensitive Skin	3 to 9 drops	0.5% to 1% dilution
Healthy Adults	9 to 18 drops	1% to 2% dilution
Short term on area of concern	18 to 27 drops	2% to 3% dilution

For more information on dilution please see first chapter.

Diffusion: Follow the instructions that came with the diffuser. To avoid over-exposure run the diffuser for only 15 to 20 minutes.

Direct Inhalation: Add a few drops to a handkerchief, tissue or cotton ball and inhale the aroma of the oil. If you choose to inhale the aroma directly from the bottle, hold the bottle a few inches below your nose and take a quick sniff or two. Be careful not to ingest the oil through your nose as that can be toxic.

References

4. http://www.britannica.com/EBchecked/topic/217294/frankincense
5. Davis, Patricia, and Sarah Budd. Aromatherapy an A-Z. London: Vermillion, 2005. Print. Page 124
6. Chemical composition and antimicrobial activity of some oleogum resin essential oils from Boswellia spp. (Burseraceae).
   Camarda L, Dayton T, Di Stefano V, Pitonzo R, Schillaci D.
   Ann Chim. 2007 Sep;97(9):837-44.
   PMID: 17970299
7. [Effects of aroma hand massage on pain, state anxiety and depression in hospice patients with terminal cancer].
   Chang SY.
   Taehan Kanho Hakhoe Chi. 2008 Aug;38(4):493-502. Korean.
   PMID:18753801
8. Tisserand, Robert and Rodney Young. *Essential Oil Safety: A Guide for Health Care Professionals*. 2nd Edition. Edinburgh: Churchill Livingston Elsevier Health Sciences. 2014. Print. Page 288

Chapter 8

Geranium

Pelargonium graveolens

Botanical Family: Geraniaceae

Parts Used: Flower

Country of Origin: Egypt

Extraction Method: Steam Distillation

History and Traditional Use

It is believed that scented geraniums (*Pelargonium*) originated in South Afri
and were brought to Europe by sailors in the early 1600s. Delightfully fragra
they were enjoyed as house plants. Medicinally they were used as treatment f
stomach ailments and astringents for wound care. A type of vinegar made w
geraniums was applied to the forehead as a headache remedy. Their great
commercial success was in the perfume industry. Geranium oil from a rose-scent
variety was used in the mid-1800s as a substitute for more expensive rose oil
geranium extract from *Pelargonium sidoides* is currently used in an over-the-coun
cold and flu preparation.[69]

Research

Antibacterial: A blend of grapefruit seed extract and geranium oil had t
most anti-bacterial activity against MRSA, and a combination of geranium and t
tree oil was most effective against methicillin-sensitive S. aureus.[70]

Antibacterial—Hard-to-Heal Wounds: Geranium essential oil was effect
against Gram-negative bacteria. The bacteria used in the study was obtained fro
patients with hard-to-heal wounds.[71]

Antibacterial—Air Disinfectant: In a laboratory-conducted study gerani
and lemongrass essential oils were tested, both as single oils and as combined o
The oils were applied on surfaces and also diffused. The results showed that t
essential oils reduced levels of antibiotic-sensitive and antibiotic-resistant bacte
from the air and surfaces.[72]

Antimicrobial: Black pepper, clove, geranium, nutmeg, oregano, and thy
essential oils were examined for antibacterial activity against twenty-five differ

kinds of bacteria. The oils were effective against all tested organisms. This included bacteria that affect plants and animals and cause food poisoning and food spoilage.[73]

Candida: Geranium essential oil (*Pelargonium graveolens*) in combination with Amphotericin B (a potent antifungal medication) appears to be most effective against all the Candida species used in this study.[74]

Insect Repellent–Paper Wasps and Yellow Jackets: A blend of clove, geranium and lemongrass oils, and also a blend of clove, geranium, lemongrass and rosemary oils totally blocked the attraction of wasps, yellow jackets and hornets.[75]

Insect Repellent–Tick Repellent: An effective insect repellent against the lone star tick, a tick that is spreading to more parts of the United States, was found in a compound isolated from geranium essential oil.[76]

Safety Tips

* Do not take geranium oil by mouth.

How To Use

To use on skin: To make your desired dilution add drops to 30 ml carrier oil and shake or mix well. Use a glass container and an accurate measuring device, not silverware.

30 ml is the equivalent of 1 ounce or 2 tablespoons or 6 teaspoons

Elderly, Frail, Sensitive Skin	3 to 9 drops	0.5% to 1% dilution
Healthy Adults	9 to 18 drops	1% to 2% dilution
Short term on area of concern	18 to 27 drops	2% to 3% dilution

For more information on dilution please see first chapter.

Diffusion: Follow the instructions that came with the diffuser. To avoid over-exposure run the diffuser for only 15 to 20 minutes.

Direct Inhalation: Add a few drops to a handkerchief, tissue or cotton ball and inhale the aroma of the oil. If you choose to inhale the aroma directly from the bottle, hold the bottle a few inches below your nose and take a quick sniff or two. Be careful not to ingest the oil through your nose as that can be toxic.

Insect spray: For immediate use make a spray with water and a few drops of geranium oil and if desired other insect-repelling essential oils such as clove, lemongrass, peppermint, rosemary, cedarwood, patchouli, orange, or ylang ylang.

Room Spray: Combine in a glass spray bottle or plant mister: 4 tablespoons distilled water, 2 tablespoons vodka and 20 to 30 drops of desired essential oils. Shake well before each use.

References

69. Kowalchik, Claire and William H. Hylton. Rodale's Illustrated Encyclopedia of Herbs. Emmaus, PA: Rodale Press, 1987. Print. Pages 455-456

70. The effect of essential oils on methicillin-resistant Staphylococcus aureus using a dressing model.
    Edwards-Jones V, Buck R, Shawcross SG, Dawson MM, Dunn K.
    Burns. 2004 Dec;30(8):772-7.
    PMID:15555788

71. The antibacterial activity of geranium oil against Gram-negative bacteria isolated from difficult-to-heal wounds.
    Sienkiewicz M, Poznańska-Kurowska K, Kaszuba A, Kowalczyk E.
    Burns. 2014 Aug;40(5):1046-51. doi: 10.1016/j.burns.2013.11.002. Epub 2013 Nov 28.
    PMID:24290961

72. Vapour-phase activities of essential oils against antibiotic sensitive and resistant bacteria including MRSA.
    Doran AL, Morden WE, Dunn K, Edwards-Jones V.
    Lett Appl Microbiol. 2009 Apr;48(4):387-92. doi: 10.1111/j.1472-765X.2009.02552.x.
    PMID:19292822

73. Antimicrobial agents from plants: antibacterial activity of plant volatile oils.
    Dorman HJ, Deans SG.
    J Appl Microbiol. 2000 Feb;88(2):308-16.
    PMID:10736000

74. The inhibition of Candida species by selected essential oils and their synergism with amphotericin B.
    Rosato A, Vitali C, Gallo D, Balenzano L, Mallamaci R.
    Phytomedicine. 2008 Aug;15(8):635-8. doi: 10.1016/j.phymed.2008.05.001. Epub 2008 Jun 24.
    PMID:18579358

75. Essential oils and their compositions as spatial repellents for pestiferous social wasps.
    Zhang QH, Schneidmiller RG, Hoover DR.
    Pest Manag Sci. 2013 Apr;69(4):542-52. doi: 10.1002/ps.3411. Epub 2012 Oct 19.
    PMID: 23081867

76. Bioactivity-guided investigation of geranium essential oils as natural tick repellents.
    Tabanca N, Wang M, Avonto C, Chittiboyina AG, Parcher JF, Carroll JF, Kramer M, Khan IA.
    J Agric Food Chem. 2013 May 1;61(17):4101-7. doi: 10.1021/jf400246a. Epub 2013 Apr 22.
    PMID:23528036

Chapter 9

Grapefruit

Citrus x paradisi

Botanical Family: Hybrid (*C. maxima* and *C.sinensis*)   **Country of Origin:** United States

Parts Used: Peel   **Extraction Method:** Cold Pressed

History and Traditional Uses

Grapefruits were discovered in Barbados in the 18th century. They are believed to be a natural cross between an orange and pomelo. The fruit hangs in clusters like grapes, hence the name grapefruit. Grapefruits are rich in vitamin C, Vitamin A, fiber and antioxidants. The grapefruit scent has been described as refreshing and stimulating. They have been used in the diet for weight loss and to reduce cholesterol.[77]

Grapefruits contain a compound (furanocoumarin) that reduces the enzymes (cytochrome P450) needed to metabolize many medications including statins. Individuals taking certain prescription medications are often advised not to eat grapefruits, or drink grapefruit juice, because the combination can cause blood levels of some medications to rise causing increased risks and side effects.[78]

Grapefruit essential oil is not likely to cause an interaction with medications because it does not contain the principle furanocoumarin responsible for causing drug interactions.[79]

Research

Anti-Aging–Skincare: This laboratory-conducted study looked at how massage with essential oils might reduce elastase, an enzyme that contributes to wrinkle formation. Elastase activity was inhibited by lemon, juniper and grapefruit essential oils.[80]

Mood–Stimulating: Inhalation of pepper oil, estragon oil (tarragon oil), fennel oil or grapefruit oil had a stimulating effect on sympathetic activity (has to do with heart rate, blood pressure). Inhalation of rose oil or patchouli oil caused a 40% decrease in relative sympathetic activity (calming effect).[81]

Tick Repellent: Nootkatone derived from grapefruit oil was found to be toxic to four tick species.[82]

Weight Loss: Researchers noted that rats exposed to the scent of grapefruit oil for fifteen minutes three times a week had less appetites and lost weight.[83]

Weight Loss: This study demonstrated that the scent of grapefruit and lemon oil increased lipolysis (the breakdown of fat) and suppressed body weight in rats.[84]

Weight Loss—Body Fat Reduction: In this study a group of post-menopausal women received a weekly one-hour whole body massage with 3% grapefruit oil, cypress oil and three other oils for six weeks. The women also massaged their own abdomens twice a day, five days a week for six weeks. The results showed significant reduction of abdominal subcutaneous fat and waist circumference.[85]

Safety Tips

- Do not take grapefruit oil by mouth.
- Always use diluted.
- Avoid sun or tanning bed exposure for 12 hours after using grapefruit essential oil on skin. Grapefruit oil is known to intensify the effects of UV light.
- Old or oxidized (rancid) oils should be avoided. Grapefruit oil should be kept in a refrigerator, stored in a dark airtight container. Tisserand and Young recommend no more than 30ml (6 teaspoons) of a 4% dilution be used on the skin per day.[86]

How To Use

To use on skin: To make your desired dilution add drops to 30 ml carrier oil and shake or mix well. Use a glass container and an accurate measuring device, not silverware.

30 ml is the equivalent of 1 ounce or 2 tablespoons or 6 teaspoons

Elderly, Frail, Sensitive Skin	3 to 9 drops	0.5% to 1% dilution
Healthy Adults	9 to 18 drops	1% to 2% dilution
Short term on area of concern	18 to 27 drops	2% to 3% dilution

For more information on dilution please see first chapter.

Diffusion: Follow the instructions that came with the diffuser. To avoid over-exposure run the diffuser for only 15 to 20 minutes.

Direct Inhalation: Add a few drops to a handkerchief, tissue or cotton ball and inhale the aroma of the oil. If you choose to inhale the aroma directly from the bottle, hold the bottle a few inches below your nose and take a quick sniff or two. Be careful not to ingest the oil through your nose as that can be toxic.

Insect Repellent: For immediate use make a spray with water and a few drops grapefruit oil and if desired other insect-repelling essential oils such as geranium, mongrass, clove, peppermint, cedarwood, patchouli, or ylang ylang.

Room Spray: Combine in a glass spray bottle or plant mister: 4 tablespoons stilled water, 2 tablespoons vodka and 20 to 30 drops of desired essential oil. ake well before each use.

Laundry: Add a few drops to laundry.

eferences

http://www.whfoods.com/genpage.php?tname=foodspice&dbid=25

http://www.drugs.com/article/grapefruit-drug-interactions.html

Tisserand, Robert and Rodney Young. *Essential Oil Safety: A Guide for Health Care Professionals*. 2nd Edition. Edinburgh: Churchill Livingston Elsevier Health Sciences. 2014. Print. Page 298

Inhibition of elastase activity by essential oils in vitro.
Mori M, Ikeda N, Kato Y, Minamino M, Watabe K.
J Cosmet Dermatol. 2002 Dec;1(4):183-7.
PMID:17147537

Effects of fragrance inhalation on sympathetic activity in normal adults.
Haze S, Sakai K, Gozu Y.
Jpn J Pharmacol. 2002 Nov;90(3):247-53.
PMID:12499579

Susceptibility of four tick species, Amblyomma americanum, Dermacentor variabilis, Ixodes scapularis, and Rhipicephalus sanguineus (Acari: Ixodidae), to nootkatone from essential oil ofgrapefruit.
Flor-Weiler LB, Behle RW, Stafford KC 3rd.
J Med Entomol. 2011 Mar;48(2):322-6.
PMID:21485368

Olfactory stimulation with scent of grapefruit oil affects autonomic nerves, lipolysis and appetite in rats.
Shen J, Niijima A, Tanida M, Horii Y, Maeda K, Nagai K.
Neurosci Lett. 2005 Jun 3;380(3):289-94. Epub 2005 Feb 5.
PMID:15862904

Effect of olfactory stimulation with flavor of grapefruit oil and lemon oil on the activity of sympathetic branch in the white adipose tissue of the epididymis.
Niijima A, Nagai K.
Exp Biol Med (Maywood). 2003 Nov;228(10):1190-2.
PMID:14610259

[Effect of aromatherapy massage on abdominal fat and body image in post-menopausal women].
Kim HJ.
Taehan Kanho Hakhoe Chi. 2007 Jun;37(4):603-12. Korean.
PMID:17615482

Tisserand, Robert and Rodney Young. E*ssential Oil Safety: A Guide for Health Care Professionals*. 2nd Edition. Edinburgh: Churchill Livingston Elsevier Health Sciences. 2014. Print. Page 297

Chapter 10

Jasmine Absolute
Absoluteum grandiflorum

〰️

Botanical Family: Oleaceae   **Country of Origin:**   India

Parts Used: Flower   **Extraction Method**:   Extraction

History and Traditional Use

Jasmine flowers are gathered at night when they are most fragrant. It take a huge amount of flowers to make a small amount of oil. The whole process expensive and labor intensive. Fortunately very little jasmine oil is needed per use.

Most essential oils are extracted by steam distillation or cold-pressed. Th flowers of jasmine are so delicate that, in order to capture their scent, a solvent used to pull the scented oil from the flowers. The final extraction produces absolu oil, which is more concentrated than essential oils.[88]

Research

Mood: Inhaled jasmine absolute has been shown to be stimulating both i animals and humans.[89]

Mood: In this study the odors of jasmine tea and lavender essential oil cause decreases in heart rate and created a calm and yet energized mood.[90]

Safety Tips

- Do not take Jasmine Absolute by mouth.
- Use caution if you have sensitive or damaged skin.
- Tisserand and Young recommend no more than 30ml (6 teaspoons) of a 0.7% dilution be used on the skin per day. Jasmine oil is a known skin sensitizer.[91]

If used too frequently on skin without enough dilution, or on skin that is damaged jasmine absolute can trigger the immune system to identify the oil as harmful an cause an allergy-like inflammatory reaction. This reaction is more common i persons who tend to have allergies.

How To Use

To use on skin: In a glass container combine carrier oil with the amount of drops needed for your desired dilution.

- To make a 0.7% dilution add 6 drops to 30ml (6 teaspoons) carrier oil.
- Jasmine is so fragrant; most persons use only a tiny amount.
- To make a small amount of 0.7% dilution combine 1 teaspoon carrier oil with 1 drop of jasmine oil.
- Use a tiny bit as perfume.

References

37. http://www.newworldencyclopedia.org/entry/Jasmine

38. https://www.naha.org/explore-aromatherapy/about-aromatherapy/how-are-essential-oils-extracted/

39. Jasmine absolute (Jasminum grandiflora L) and its mode of action on guinea-pig ileum in vitro.
Lis-Balchin M, Hart S, Wan Hang Lo B.
Phytother Res. 2002 Aug;16(5):437-9.
PMID:12203263

40. Sedative effects of the jasmine tea odor and (R)-(-)-linalool, one of its major odor components, on autonomic nerve activity and mood states.
Kuroda K, Inoue N, Ito Y, Kubota K, Sugimoto A, Kakuda T, Fushiki T.
Eur J Appl Physiol. 2005 Oct;95(2-3):107-14. Epub 2005 Jun 23.
PMID:15976995

41. Tisserand, Robert and Rodney Young. *Essential Oil Safety: A Guide for Health Care Professionals.* 2nd Edition. Edinburgh: Churchill Livingston Elsevier HealthSciences. 2014. Print. Page 312

Chapter 11

Lavender

Lavandula angustifolia

❧

Botanical Family: Lamiaceae (mint)   **Country of Origin**:   France and Bulgaria

Parts Used: Flower and Stem   **Extraction Method**:   Steam Distillation

History and Traditional Uses

Lavender was highly valued throughout the ancient world. It was used f
bathing, to relieve headaches, to heal and disinfect burns and wounds, and as an a
freshener, insect repellent and for bathing.[92]

Lavender essential oil is one of the most useful oils. According to Patricia Dav
author of *Aromatherapy an A-Z*, lavender's chemical structure makes it useful as a
analgesic, antidepressant, antiseptic, antibacterial, decongestant, sedative, and hel
repel insects. It is also useful in the treatment of colds, coughs and sinusitis.[93]

Research

Alzheimer's disease and Dementia: Significant improvement was seen
cognitive function by using aromatherapy with rosemary and lemon essential o
in the morning, and lavender and orange essential oils in the evening.[94]

Anti-inflammatory, Anti-aging: This study found that inhalation of lavend
and rosemary essential oils improved the body's free radical scavenging abilit
which in turn reduced damaging oxidative stress. Oxidative stress is recognized
a harmful factor in aging and in many diseases.[95]

Antimicrobial: Vapors of tea tree oil, bergamot, lavender and eucalypt
inhibited both bacteria and fungi.[96]

Anxiety: In this study inhalation of orange and lavender essential oils helpe
reduce anxiety.[97]

Anxiety and Depression: Topically applied blended lavender and bergam
essential oils reduced pulse rate and blood pressure. This blend may be used f
treating depression and anxiety.[98]

Anxiety–Workplace Stress: Researchers had one group of nurses pin sm bottles containing 3% lavender oil on their chest. Their stress symptoms significantly decreased while stress symptoms increased in the control group.[99]

Arthritis: Using a blend of lavender, marjoram, eucalyptus, rosemary, and peppermint oils diluted in carrier oil significantly lowered arthritic pain and depression.[100]

Blood Pressure–Stress: Researchers found that persons with essential hypertension who inhaled a combination of lavender, ylang ylang and bergamot essential oils once daily were able to reduce psychological stress as well as blood pressure.[101]

Blood Pressure: In this study prehypertensive and hypertensive subjects inhaled a blended combination of lavender, ylang ylang, marjoram and neroli. Daytime blood pressure readings were significantly reduced and subjects were more relaxed than the placebo and control groups.[102]

Hair Growth–Alopecia Areata: In this study one group massaged thyme, rosemary, lavender and cedarwood essential oils mixed with carrier oil on their scalp. The other group massaged with only carrier oil. Forty-three percent of the patients massaging the essential oils on their scalp showed improvement versus 15% improvement in the carrier oil group.[103]

Hospice Care: Aromatherapy hand massage was beneficial for reducing pain and depression in hospice patients with terminal cancer. Each hand was massaged for five minutes with a blended mixture of bergamot, lavender and frankincense essential oils.[104]

Insect Repellent: Lavender, myrtle and salvia essential oils were found to be effective insect repellents at 10% concentration.[105]

Insect Repellent–Ticks: For repelling ticks, lavender oil compared well to DEET.[106]

Insomnia and Depression: Researchers tested lavender fragrance on forty-two women (college students) suffering from insomnia, and found that lavender fragrance reduced insomnia and depression.[107]

Insomnia: This study looked at how lavender aromatherapy affects both men and women. Researchers found that lavender aromatherapy increased deep sleep in men and women. Everyone who used lavender essential oil felt more energized the next morning.[108]

Menstrual Pain: Duration of menstrual pain was reduced by massaging a blend of lavender, clary sage and marjoram essential oils to the lower abdomen. The patients applied the essential oils every day from the last day of their period to the beginning of the next period.[109]

Menstrual Pain: In this study menstrual pain was reduced by lavender oil massage. The lavender oil was applied at the start of menstruation.[110]

Menstrual Pain: Massaging the abdomen with cinnamon, clove, rose, and lavender in carrier oil for seven days, before menstruation, alleviated menstrual pain and reduced the amount of menstrual bleeding.[111]

Migraine Headache: This study found that inhalation of lavender essential oil may be used to treat migraines.[112]

Pain—After Tonsillectomy: Researchers treated twenty-four children with lavender aromatherapy and acetaminophen, and treated twenty-four children with only acetaminophen. The children that received aromatherapy with lavender and acetaminophen used less acetaminophen than the children who did not receive lavender essential oil aromatherapy.[113]

Premenstrual Syndrome: Many women suffer monthly from dreaded PMS symptoms such as mood swings, food cravings, headaches, fatigue, anxiety, irritability, depression and changes in sleep patterns. Lavender aromatherapy can relieve premenstrual symptoms.[114]

Safety Tips

Lavender has been safely used and held dear for thousands of years. It is considered safe and non-toxic. It is often used neat on an insect sting, bite or sore. Persons who tend to have allergies or very sensitive skin should dilute lavender oil.

*   Do not take by mouth.
*   Dilute for use on skin especially if you tend to be allergic.

How To Use

To use on skin: To make your desired dilution add drops to 30 ml carrier oil and shake or mix well. Use a glass container and an accurate measuring device not silverware.

30 ml is the equivalent of 1 ounce or 2 tablespoons or 6 teaspoons

Elderly, Frail, Sensitive Skin	3 to 9 drops	0.5% to 1% dilution
Healthy Adults	9 to 18 drops	1% to 2% dilution
Short term on area of concern	18 to 27 drops	2% to 3% dilution

For more information on dilution please see first chapter.

Bath: Add a few diluted drops to a bath

To fight a cold and get ready for bed: add 1 cup Epsom Salts to a warm bath.[216] Combine 3 drops tea tree oil, 3 drops eucalyptus oil and 3 drops lavender oil in 30ml carrier oil. (6 teaspoons) Massage on arms and legs. Relax in a warm bath.

Diffusion: Follow the instructions that came with the diffuser. To avoid over exposure run the diffuser for only 15 to 20 minutes.

Direct Inhalation: Add a few drops to a handkerchief, tissue or cotton ball and inhale the aroma of the oil. If you choose to inhale the aroma directly from the bottle, hold the bottle a few inches below your nose and take a quick sniff or two. Be careful not to ingest the oil through your nose as that can be toxic.

Insect Repellent: For immediate use, make a spray with water and a few drops of lavender oil and, if desired, other insect-repelling essential oils such as cedarwood, patchouli, geranium, peppermint, lemongrass or ylang ylang.

Room Spray: Combine in a glass spray bottle or plant mister: 4 tablespoons distilled water, 2 tablespoons vodka and 20 to 30 drops of desired essential oils. Shake well before each use.

Laundry: Add a few drops to laundry.

References

92. Hanrahan, Clare; Odle, Teresa. "Lavender." Gale Encyclopedia of Alternative Medicine. 2005 Volume 3 (Lavender) page1185-1186

93. Davis, Patricia, and Sarah Budd. *Aromatherapy an A-Z*. London:Vermillion, 2005. Print. Page 176-177

94. 94. Effect of aromatherapy on patients with Alzheimer's disease.
Jimbo D, Kimura Y, Taniguchi M, Inoue M, Urakami K.
Psychogeriatrics. 2009 Dec;9(4):173-9. doi: 10.1111/j.1479-8301.2009.00299.x.
PMID:20377818

95. Smelling lavender and rosemary increases free radical scavenging activity and decreases cortisol level in saliva.
Atsumi T, Tonosaki K.
Psychiatry Res. 2007 Feb 28;150(1):89-96. Epub 2007 Feb 7.
PMID:17291597

96. Vapour phase: a potential future use for essential oils as antimicrobials?
Laird K, Phillips C.
Lett Appl Microbiol. 2012 Mar;54(3):169-74. doi: 10.1111/j.1472-765X.2011.03190.x. Epub 2012 Jan 6.
PMID:22133088

97. Ambient odors of orange and lavender reduce anxiety and improve mood in a dental office.
Lehrner J, Marwinski G, Lehr S, Johren P, Deecke L.
Physiol Behav. 2005 Sep 15;86(1-2):92-5.
PMID:16095639

98. Aroma-therapeutic effects of massage blended essential oils on humans.
Hongratanaworakit T.
Nat Prod Commun. 2011 Aug;6(8):1199-204.
PMID:21922934

99. The effects of aromatherapy in relieving symptoms related to job stress among nurses.
Chen MC, Fang SH, Fang L.
Int J Nurs Pract. 2015 Feb;21(1):87-93. doi: 10.1111/ijn.12229. Epub 2013 Nov 15.
PMID: 24238073

00. [The effects of aromatherapy on pain, depression, and life satisfaction of arthritis patients].
Kim MJ, Nam ES, Paik SI.
Taehan Kanho Hakhoe Chi. 2005 Feb;35(1):186-94. Korean.
PMID: 15778570

01. [The effects of the inhalation method using essential oils on blood pressure and stress responses of clients with essential hypertension].
Hwang JH.
Taehan Kanho Hakhoe Chi. 2006 Dec;36(7):1123-34. Korean.
PMID:17211115

102. Essential oil inhalation on blood pressure and salivary cortisol levels in prehypertensive and hypertensive subjects.
Kim IH, Kim C, Seong K, Hur MH, Lim HM, Lee MS.

103. Randomized trial of aromatherapy. Successful treatment for alopecia areata.
Hay IC, Jamieson M, Ormerod AD.
Arch Dermatol. 1998 Nov;134(11):1349-52.
PMID:9828867

104. [Effects of aroma hand massage on pain, state anxiety and depression in hospice patients with terminal cancer].
Chang SY.
Taehan Kanho Hakhoe Chi. 2008 Aug;38(4):493-502. Korean.
PMID:18753801

105. Evaluation of Repellency Effect of Essential Oils of Satureja khuzestanica (Carvacrol), Myrtus communis (Myrtle), Lavendula officinalis and Salvia sclarea using Standard WHO Repellency Tests.
Kayedi MH, Haghdoost AA, Salehnia A, Khamisabadi K.
J Arthropod Borne Dis. 2013 Dec 18;8(1):60-8. eCollection 2014.
PMID: 25629066

106. Repellent effects of the essential oil of Lavendula angustifolia against adults of Hyalomma marginatum rufipes.
Mkolo MN, Magano SR.
J S Afr Vet Assoc. 2007 Sep;78(3):149-52.
PMID:18237038

107. Effects of lavender aromatherapy on insomnia and depression in women college students].
Lee IS, Lee GJ.
Taehan Kanho Hakhoe Chi. 2006 Feb;36(1):136-43. Korean.
PMID:16520572.

108. An olfactory stimulus modifies nighttime sleep in young men and women.
Goel N, Kim H, Lao RP.
Chronobiol Int. 2005;22(5):889-904.
PMID: 16298774

109. Pain relief assessment by aromatic essential oil massage on outpatients with primary dysmenorrhea: a randomized, double-blind clinical trial.
Ou MC, Hsu TF, Lai AC, Lin YT, Lin CC.
J Obstet Gynaecol Res. 2012 May;38(5):817-22. doi: 10.1111/j.1447-0756.2011.01802.x. Epub 2012 Mar 22.
PMID: 22435409

110. The effect of aromatherapy massage with lavender oil on severity of primary dysmenorrhea in Arsanjan students.
Bakhtshirin F, Abedi S, YusefiZoj P, Razmjooee D.
Iran J Nurs Midwifery Res. 2015 Jan-Feb;20(1):156-60.
PMID:25709705

111. The effect of aromatherapy abdominal massage on alleviating menstrual pain in nursing students: a prospective randomized cross-over study.
Marzouk TM, El-Nemer AM, Baraka HN.
Evid Based Complement Alternat Med. 2013;2013:742421. doi: 10.1155/2013/742421. Epub 2013 Apr 11.
PMID:23662151

112. Lavender essential oil in the treatment of migraine headache: a placebo-controlled clinical trial.
Sasannejad P, Saeedi M, Shoeibi A, Gorji A, Abbasi M, Foroughipour M.
Eur Neurol. 2012;67(5):288-91. doi: 10.1159/000335249. Epub 2012 Apr 17.
PMID:22517298

3. Evaluation of the effect of aromatherapy with lavender essential oil on post-tonsillectomy pain in pediatric patients: a randomized controlled trial.
Soltani R, Soheilipour S, Hajhashemi V, Asghari G, Bagheri M, Molavi M.
Int J Pediatr Otorhinolaryngol. 2013 Sep;77(9):1579-81. doi: 10.1016/j.ijporl.2013.07.014. Epub 2013 Aug 8.
PMID:23932834

4. Does lavender aromatherapy alleviate premenstrual emotional symptoms?: a randomized crossover trial.
Matsumoto T, Asakura H, Hayashi T.
Biopsychosoc Med. 2013 May 31;7:12. doi: 10.1186/1751-0759-7-12. eCollection 2013.
PMID:23724853

5. http://www.epsomsaltcouncil.org/news/articles/doctors_say_treat_colds_flu_with_epsom_salt.php

Chapter 12

Lemon
Citrus limon

~~~

Botanical Family:	Rutaceae	**Country of Origin**:	Argentina
Parts Used:	Peel	**Extraction Method**:	Cold Pressed

History and Traditional Uses

The lovely lemon tree can produce fragrant blooms several times a year and unlike other citrus varieties, it can produce fruit continuously. In the 1600s physician realized that citrus fruits prevented scurvy. Later scientists determined that it wa the vitamin C that kept the sailors healthy during long sea voyages.[116]

Research

Alzheimer's disease and Dementia: Significant improvement was seen i cognitive function by using aromatherapy with rosemary and lemon essential oi in the morning, and lavender and orange essential oils in the evening.[117]

Anti-Aging–Skin: This laboratory-conducted study looked at how massag with essential oils might reduce elastase, an enzyme that contributes to wrin kle formation. Elastase activity was inhibited by lemon, juniper and grapefru essential oils.[118]

Antimicrobial: Essentials oils were demonstrated by laboratory testing to b an inexpensive and effective option for treatment of hospital acquired, antibiotic resistant, and common strains of bacteria, including MRSA and antimycotic resisitant Candida species. The most effective of the tested oils were: white thyme lemon, lemongrass and cinnamon oil.[119]

Constipation: Abdominal massage with a blend of rosemary, lemon and peppermint oils helped relieve constipation.[120]

Depression and Immune Stimulating: Researchers explain that inhalation c a citrus fragrance can repair stress-caused immunosuppression. They also explai that depressed patients who inhaled a citrus fragrance were able to use much les medication to treat their depression.[121]

Morning Sickness—Pregnancy: Researchers found that inhalation of lemon oil can be effective in reducing nausea and vomiting when pregnant.[122]

Weight Loss: This study demonstrated that the scent of grapefruit and lemon oil increased lipolysis, the breakdown of fat, and suppressed body weight in rats.[123]

Safety Tips

- Do not take lemon oil by mouth.
- Always use diluted.
- Avoid sun or tanning bed exposure for 12 hours after using lemon essential oil on the skin. Lemon oil can intensify the effects of UV light.

Tisserand and Young recommend no more than 30ml (6 teaspoons) of a 2% dilution be used on the skin per day.

They also suggest that old or oxidized oils be avoided. Lemon oil should be kept in the refrigerator, stored in a dark airtight container.[124]

How To Use

To use on skin: In a glass container combine carrier oil with the amount of drops needed for your desired dilution.

- To make a 1% dilution add 9 drops to 30ml carrier oil (6 teaspoons)
- To make a 2% dilution add 18 drops to 30ml carrier oil (6 teaspoons)

Diffusion: Follow the instructions that came with the diffuser. To avoid over-exposure run the diffuser for only 15 to 20 minutes.

Direct Inhalation: Add a few drops to a handkerchief, tissue or cotton ball and inhale the aroma of the oil. If you choose to inhale the aroma directly from the bottle, hold the bottle a few inches below your nose and take a quick sniff or two. Be careful not to ingest the oil through your nose as that can be toxic.

Room Spray: Combine in a glass-spray bottle or plant mister: 4 tablespoons distilled water, 2 tablespoons vodka and 20 to 30 drops of desired essential oils. Shake well before each use.

Laundry: Add a few drops to laundry.

References

6. http://www.drugs.com/npp/lemon.html

7. Effect of aromatherapy on patients with Alzheimer's disease.
    Jimbo D, Kimura Y, Taniguchi M, Inoue M, Urakami K.
    Psychogeriatrics. 2009 Dec;9(4):173-9. doi: 10.1111/j.1479-8301.2009.00299.x.
    PMID:20377818

8. Inhibition of elastase activity by essential oils in vitro.
    Mori M, Ikeda N, Kato Y, Minamino M, Watabe K.
    J Cosmet Dermatol. 2002 Dec;1(4):183-7.
    PMID:17147537

119. The battle against multi-resistant strains: Renaissance of antimicrobial essential oils as a promising force to fight hospital-acquired infections.
Warnke PH, Becker ST, Podschun R, Sivananthan S, Springer IN, Russo PA, Wiltfang J, Fickenscher H, Sherry E.
J Craniomaxillofac Surg. 2009 Oct;37(7):392-7. doi: 10.1016/j.jcms.2009.03.017. Epub 2009 May 20
PMID:19473851

120. [Effect of aromatherapy massage for the relief of constipation in the elderly].
Kim MA, Sakong JK, Kim EJ, Kim EH, Kim EH.
Taehan Kanho Hakhoe Chi. 2005 Feb;35(1):56-64. Korean.
PMID:15778557

121. Effects of citrus fragrance on immune function and depressive states.
Komori T, Fujiwara R, Tanida M, Nomura J, Yokoyama MM.
Neuroimmunomodulation. 1995 May-Jun;2(3):174-80.
PMID:8646568

122. The effect of lemon inhalation aromatherapy on nausea and vomiting of pregnancy: a double-blinded, randomized, controlled clinical trial.
Yavari Kia P, Safajou F, Shahnazi M, Nazemiyeh H.

123. Effect of olfactory stimulation with flavor of grapefruit oil and lemon oil on the activity of sympathetic branch in the white adipose tissue of the epididymis.
Niijima A, Nagai K.
Exp Biol Med (Maywood). 2003 Nov;228(10):1190-2.
PMID:14610259

124. Tisserand, Robert and Rodney Young. *Essential Oil Safety: A Guide for Health Care Professionals.* 2nd Edition. Edinburgh: Churchill Livingston Elsevier Health Sciences. 2014. Print. Page 331

Chapter 13

Lemongrass
Cymbopogon flexuosus

Botanical Family:	Poaceae (Grass)		**Country of Origin**:	Guatemala
Parts Used:	Leaf, Stem		**Extraction Method**:	Steam Distillation

History and Traditional Use

Lemongrass is a perennial herb grown in the tropics. *Cymbopogon flexuosus* is known as East Indian lemongrass and is said to have antifungal and insect-repellent activity. Its main chemical constituent is citral.[125]

Research

Antibacterial–Air Disinfectant: In a laboratory-conducted study geranium and lemongrass essential oils were tested, both as single oils and as combined oils. The oils were applied on surfaces and diffused into the air. The results showed that the essential oils reduced levels of antibiotic-sensitive and antibiotic-resistant bacteria from the air and on surfaces.[126]

Antibacterial–Hospital Acquired Infections: Lemongrass was found to be very effective against Gram-positive bacteria, and tea tree oil was very effective against Gram-negative bacteria. Antiseptic essential oils are showing strong potential as affordable topical treatments to prevent multi-resistant, hospital-acquired infections.[127]

Antibacterial–Respiratory Infections: 14 essential oils were tested against bacteria that cause respiratory infection. Thyme, cinnamon bark, lemongrass, perilla, and peppermint oils were found effective and chosen for further evaluation.[128]

Antifungal–Candida albicans: Oregano, winter savory, peppermint, cinnamon bark and lemongrass showed the most activity against Candida albicans.[129]

Antimicrobial: In a laboratory-conducted study lemongrass showed the most antimicrobial and anti-biofilm activity against five strains of Staphylococcus aureus.[130]

Insect Repellent: Essential oils have been investigated for use as natural insect and arthropod repellents. (Ants, bed bugs, fleas, house flies, ticks and mosquitoes are arthropods.) Monoterpenes and sesquiterpenes appear to be insect-repelling compounds. Lemongrass, basil and eucalyptus essential oils contain compounds that are most noted as effective insect repellents.[131]

Insect Repellent–Paper Wasps and Yellow Jackets: A blend of clove, geranium and lemongrass oils, and also a blend of clove, geranium, lemongrass and rosemary oils totally blocked the attraction of wasps, yellow jackets and hornets.[132]

Safety Tips

- Do not take lemongrass essential oil by mouth.
- Do not use if pregnant or nursing.
- Do not use on children under 2 years old.
- Use caution if you have sensitive or damaged skin.
- Tisserand and Young recommend no more than 30ml (6 teaspoons) of a 0.7% dilution be used on the skin per day.[133]

How To Use

To use on skin: In a glass container combine the amount of carrier oil with the amount of drops needed for your desired dilution.

- To make a 0.7% dilution add 6 drops to 30ml (6 teaspoons) carrier oil.
- To make a smaller amount of a 0.7% dilution add 1 drop to 1 teaspoon (5ml) carrier oil.

Diffusing: To reduce airborne-microbes, diffuse lemongrass oil for a few minutes in a well-ventilated room. Note the safety concern for young children and if pregnant.

Insect Repellent: For immediate use make a spray with water and a few drops of lemongrass and, if desired, other insect-repelling essential oils such as peppermint, cedarwood, patchouli, geranium, lavender, rosemary or ylang ylang.

References

125. http://www.hort.purdue.edu/newcrop/med-aro/factsheets/lemongrass.html

126. Vapour-phase activities of essential oils against antibiotic sensitive and resistant bacteria including MRSA.
    Doran AL, Morden WE, Dunn K, Edwards-Jones V.
    Lett Appl Microbiol. 2009 Apr;48(4):387-92. doi: 10.1111/j.1472-765X.2009.02552.x.
    PMID:19292822

127. The ongoing battle against multi-resistant strains: in-vitro inhibition of hospital-acquired MRSA, VRE, Pseudomonas, ESBL E. coli and Klebsiella species in the presence of plant-derived antiseptic oils.
    Warnke PH, Lott AJ, Sherry E, Wiltfang J, Podschun R.
    J Craniomaxillofac Surg. 2013 Jun;41(4):321-6. doi: 10.1016/j.jcms.2012.10.012. Epub 2012 Nov 29.
    PMID:23199627

128. Screening of the antibacterial effects of a variety of essential oils on respiratory tract pathogens, using a modified dilution assay method.
Inouye S, Yamaguchi H, Takizawa T.
J Infect Chemother. 2001 Dec;7(4):251-4.
PMID:11810593

29. The inhibition of Candida albicans by selected essential oils and their major components.
Tampieri MP, Galuppi R, Macchioni F, Carelle MS, Falcioni L, Cioni PL, Morelli I.
Mycopathologia. 2005 Apr;159(3):339-45.
PMID:15883716

30. The anti-biofilm activity of lemongrass (Cymbopogon flexuosus) and grapefruit (Citrus paradisi)essential oils against five strains of Staphylococcus aureus.
Adukwu EC, Allen SC, Phillips CA.
J Appl Microbiol. 2012 Nov;113(5):1217-27. doi: 10.1111/j.1365-2672.2012.05418.x. Epub 2012 Aug 21.
PMID:22862808

31. Repellent activity of essential oils: a review.
Nerio LS, Olivero-Verbel J, Stashenko E.
Bioresour Technol. 2010 Jan;101(1):372-8. doi: 10.1016/j.biortech.2009.07.048. Epub 2009 Sep 2.
Review.
PMID: 19729299

32. Essential oils and their compositions as spatial repellents for pestiferous social wasps.
Zhang QH, Schneidmiller RG, Hoover DR.
Pest Manag Sci. 2013 Apr;69(4):542-52. doi: 10.1002/ps.3411. Epub 2012 Oct 19.
PMID: 23081867

33. Tisserand, Robert and Rodney Young. *Essential Oil Safety: A Guide for Health Care Professionals.* 2nd Edition. Edinburgh: Churchill Livingston Elsevier Health Sciences. 2014. Print. Page 334

Chapter 14

Marjoram

Origanum marjorana

Botanical Family: Labiatae

Parts Used: Leaf

Country of Origin: Spain

Extraction Method: Steam Distillation

History and Traditional Use

We are most familiar with marjoram as a cooking spice. Early Greek and Romans used marjoram for muscle and joint pains. It was also used to reduce the pain of menstrual cramps, headaches, and as a sleeping aid.[134]

Research

Arthritis: Using a blend of lavender, marjoram, eucalyptus, rosemary, and peppermint oils in carrier oil significantly lowered pain and depression.[135]

Blood Pressure: In this study prehypertensive and hypertensive subjects inhaled a blend of lavender, ylang ylang, marjoram and neroli. Daytime blood pressure readings were significantly reduced and subjects were more relaxed than the placebo and control groups.[136]

Menstrual Pain: Duration of menstrual pain was reduced by massaging a blend of lavender, clary sage and marjoram essential oils to the lower abdomen. The patients used the essential oils every day from the last day of their period to the beginning of the next period.[137]

Safety Tips

- Do not take by mouth.
- Do not use if pregnant or nursing.

How To Use

To use on skin: To make your desired dilution add drops to 30 ml carrier oil and shake or mix well. Use a glass container and an accurate measuring device, not silverware.

30 ml is the equivalent of 1 ounce or 2 tablespoons or 6 teaspoons

Elderly, Frail, Sensitive Skin	3 to 9 drops	0.5% to 1% dilution
Healthy Adults	9 to 18 drops	1% to 2% dilution
Short term on area of concern	18 to 27 drops	2% to 3% dilution

For more information on dilution please see first chapter.

Diffusion: Follow the instructions that came with the diffuser. To avoid overexposure run the diffuser for only 15 to 20 minutes. Note safety concern if pregnant or nursing.

Direct Inhalation: Add a few drops to a handkerchief, tissue or cotton ball and inhale the aroma of the oil. If you choose to inhale the aroma directly from the bottle, hold the bottle a few inches below your nose and take a quick sniff or two. Be careful not to ingest the oil through your nose as that can be toxic.

References

34. Castleman, Michael. *The Healing Herbs, The Ultimate Guide to the Curative Power of Natures Medicines*. Emmaus: Rodale Press, 1991. Print. Page 241

35. [The effects of aromatherapy on pain, depression, and life satisfaction of arthritis patients].
    Kim MJ, Nam ES, Paik SI.
    Taehan Kanho Hakhoe Chi. 2005 Feb;35(1):186-94. Korean.
    PMID: 15778570

36. Essential oil inhalation on blood pressure and salivary cortisol levels in prehypertensive and hypertensive subjects.
    Kim IH, Kim C, Seong K, Hur MH, Lim HM, Lee MS.
    Evid Based Complement Alternat Med. 2012;2012:984203. doi: 10.1155/2012/984203. Epub 2012 Nov 19.
    PMID:23259002

37. Pain relief assessment by aromatic essential oil massage on outpatients with primary dysmenorrhea: a randomized, double-blind clinical trial.
    Ou MC, Hsu TF, Lai AC, Lin YT, Lin CC.
    J Obstet Gynaecol Res. 2012 May;38(5):817-22. doi: 10.1111/j.1447-0756.2011.01802.x. Epub 2012 Mar 22.
    PMID: 22435409

Myrrh
Commiphora myrrha

Botanical Family: Burseraceae

Parts Used: Resin

Country of Origin: Eastern Africa

Extraction Method: Steam Distillation

History and Traditional Uses

Since ancient times, myrrh has been used for reducing pain, skin infections, inflammation, diarrhea and periodontal diseases. Myrrh has antiseptic, anesthetic and antitumor properties. The main compounds in myrrh are terpenoids, particularly furanosesquiterpenes.[138]

Research

Anti-Aging Skin Protection: This study showed that myrrh essential oil provides protection against sun damage.[139]

Antibacterial: Staphylococcus aureus can be difficult to treat. It forms biofilm, a film of bacteria that sticks to a surface. This study examined eighty-three essential oils and found that black pepper, cananga, and myrrh oils inhibited Staphylococcus aureus biofilm formation.[140]

Antimicrobial: An analysis of myrrh found considerable antimicrobial activity.[141]

Antimicrobial: Frankincense and myrrh essential oils were tested, together and individually, and found effective against a selection of pathogens. The effect was stronger when frankincense and myrrh essential oils were used together.[142]

Safety Tips

- Do not take myrrh oil by mouth.
- Do not use if pregnant or nursing.

How To Use

To use on skin: To make your desired dilution add drops to 30 ml carrier oil and shake or mix well. Use a glass container and an accurate measuring device, not silverware.

30 ml is the equivalent of 1 ounce or 2 tablespoons or 6 teaspoons

Elderly, Frail, Sensitive Skin	3 to 6 drops	0.5% to 1% dilution
Healthy Adults	9 to 18 drops	1% to 2% dilution
Short term on area of concern	18 to 27 drops	2% to 3% dilution

For more information on dilution please see first chapter.

Diffusion: Follow the instructions that came with the diffuser. To avoid over-exposure run the diffuser for only 15 to 20 minutes. Note the safety concern if pregnant or nursing

Direct Inhalation: Add a few drops to a handkerchief, tissue or cotton ball and inhale the aroma of the oil. If you choose to inhale the aroma directly from the bottle, hold the bottle a few inches below your nose and take a quick sniff or two. Be careful not to ingest the oil through your nose as that can be toxic.

References

38. Myrrh: medical marvel or myth of the Magi?
    Nomicos EY.
    Holist Nurs Pract. 2007 Nov-Dec;21(6):308-23. Review.
    PMID:17978635

39. Protection against singlet oxygen, the main actor of sebum squalene peroxidation during sun exposure, using Commiphora myrrha essential oil.
    Auffray B.
    Int J Cosmet Sci. 2007 Feb;29(1):23-9. doi: 10.1111/j.1467-2494.2007.00360.x.
    PMID:18489308

40. Anti-biofilm, anti-hemolysis, and anti-virulence activities of black pepper, cananga, myrrh oils, and nerolidol against Staphylococcus aureus.
    Lee K, Lee JH, Kim SI, Cho MH, Lee J.
    Appl Microbiol Biotechnol. 2014 Nov;98(22):9447-57. doi: 10.1007/s00253-014-5903-4. Epub 2014 Jul 16.
    PMID:25027570

41. Components, therapeutic value and uses of myrrh.
    El Ashry ES, Rashed N, Salama OM, Saleh A.
    Pharmazie. 2003 Mar;58(3):163-8. Review.
    PMID:12685809

42. The additive and synergistic antimicrobial effects of select frankincense and myrrh oils--a combination from the pharaonic pharmacopoeia.
    de Rapper S, Van Vuuren SF, Kamatou GP, Viljoen AM, Dagne E.
    Lett Appl Microbiol. 2012 Apr;54(4):352-8. doi: 10.1111/j.1472-765X.2012.03216.x. Epub 2012 Feb 20.
    PMID:22288378

Chapter 16

Orange
Citrus sinensis

Botanical Family: Rutaceae Citrus   **Country of Origin**:   United States

Parts Used: Peel   **Extraction Method**:   Cold Pressed

History and Traditional Use

The sweet orange has been cultivated since ancient times. While the fruit and juice are enjoyed as food, the essential oil is used for herbal medicine. The oil is antiseptic, anti-inflammatory and has been used for depression and stress reduction.[143]

Research

Alzheimer's Disease and Dementia: Significant improvement was seen in cognitive function by using aromatherapy with rosemary and lemon essential oils in the morning and lavender and orange essential oils in the evening.[144]

Antimicrobial–Acne: This study notes that acne-causing bacteria have developed antibiotic resistance, and that there is a need to find alternative treatments. An orange and basil essential oil formulation was found effective in the treatment of acne.[145]

Anxiety: In this study inhalation of orange and lavender essential oils helped reduce anxiety.[146]

Anxiety: Inhalation of orange essential oil helped reduce severe anxiety. Sweet orange essential oil was found to act like tranquilizer.[147]

Anxiety: Since citrus essential oils have been used for anxiety, this study looked at how diffused orange essential oil would affect children during dental treatment. The results showed reduced salivary cortisol levels and lower pulse rate indicating reduced stress.[148]

Insecticide: Orange essential oil was found to have insecticidal activity against mosquito, cockroach and housefly when used as a room spray. Cockroaches were most affected.[149]

Knee Pain: Moderate-to-severe knee pain was treated by massage with ginger and orange essential oil. There was improvement in function and reduced pain.[150]

Safety Tips

Do not take orange oil by mouth.

Do not use if pregnant or nursing.

Tisserand and Young suggest that old or oxidized oils be avoided. Orange oil should be kept in a refrigerator, stored in a dark airtight container. They also note that expressed (cold pressed) sweet orange oil does not cause phototoxicity (intensified reaction to UV light).[151]

Most citrus oils are known to cause sun sensitivity, and come with warnings to avoid sun exposure and tanning beds for twelve hours after use.

How To Use

To use on skin: To make your desired dilution add drops to 30 ml carrier oil and shake or mix well. Use a glass container and an accurate measuring device, not silverware.

30 ml is the equivalent of 1 ounce or 2 tablespoons or 6 teaspoons

Elderly, Frail, Sensitive Skin	3 to 9 drops	0.5% to 1% dilution
Healthy Adults	9 to 18 drops	1% to 2% dilution
Short term on area of concern	18 to 27 drops	2% to 3% dilution

For more information on dilution please see first chapter.

Diffusion: Follow the instructions that came with the diffuser. To avoid overexposure run the diffuser for only 15 to 20 minutes. Note the safety concern if pregnant or nursing.

Direct Inhalation: Add a few drops to a handkerchief, tissue or cotton ball and inhale the aroma of the oil. If you choose to inhale the aroma directly from the bottle, hold the bottle a few inches below your nose and take a quick sniff or two. Be careful not to ingest the oil through your nose as that can be toxic.

Insect Spray: For immediate use make a spray with water and a few drops of orange essential oil and if desired other insect-repelling essential oils such as cedarwood, patchouli, peppermint, geranium, lemongrass or ylang ylang.

Room Spray: Combine in a glass spray bottle or plant mister: 4 tablespoons distilled water, 2 tablespoons vodka and 20 to 30 drops of desired essential oils. Shake well before each use.

References

143. http://www.herbal-supplement-resource.com/sweet-orange.html

144. Effect of aromatherapy on patients with Alzheimer's disease.
Jimbo D, Kimura Y, Taniguchi M, Inoue M, Urakami K.
Psychogeriatrics. 2009 Dec;9(4):173-9. doi: 10.1111/j.1479-8301.2009.00299.x.
PMID:20377818

145. [Effectiveness of antimicrobial formulations for acne based on orange (Citrus sinensis) and sweet basil (Ocimum basilicum L) essential oils].
Matiz G, Osorio MR, Camacho F, Atencia M, Herazo J.
Biomedica. 2012 Jan-Mar;32(1):125-33. doi: 10.1590/S0120-41572012000100014. Spanish.
PMID: 23235794

146. Ambient odors of orange and lavender reduce anxiety and improve mood in a dental office.
Lehrner J, Marwinski G, Lehr S, Johren P, Deecke L.
Physiol Behav. 2005 Sep 15;86(1-2):92-5.
PMID:16095639

147. Effect of sweet orange aroma on experimental anxiety in humans.
Goes TC, Antunes FD, Alves PB, Teixeira-Silva F.
J Altern Complement Med. 2012 Aug;18(8):798-804. doi: 10.1089/acm.2011.0551. Epub 2012 Jul 31.
PMID: 22849536

148. Effect of aromatherapy with orange essential oil on salivary cortisol and pulse rate in children during dental treatment: A randomized controlled clinical trial.
Jafarzadeh M, Arman S, Pour FF.
Adv Biomed Res. 2013 Mar 6;2:10. doi: 10.4103/2277-9175.107968. Print 2013.
PMID:23930255

149. Insecticidal properties of volatile extracts of orange peels.
Ezeonu FC, Chidume GI, Udedi SC.
Bioresour Technol. 2001 Feb;76(3):273-4.
PMID:11198181

150. An experimental study on the effectiveness of massage with aromatic ginger and orange essential oil for moderate-to-severe knee pain among the elderly in Hong Kong.
Yip YB, Tam AC.
Complement Ther Med. 2008 Jun;16(3):131-8. doi: 10.1016/j.ctim.2007.12.003. Epub 2008 Mar 4.
PMID:18534325

151. Tisserand, Robert and Rodney Young. *Essential Oil Safety: A Guide for Health Care Professionals.* 2nd Edition. Edinburgh: Churchill Livingston Elsevier Health Sciences. 2014. Print. Page 372

Chapter 17

Oregano
Origanum Vulgare

Botanical Family:	Labiatae (mint)	**Country of Origin**:	Hungary
Parts Used:	Leaf	**Extraction Method**:	Steam Distillation

History and Traditional Use

We are most familiar with oregano as a spice used on pizza, but through-out history, and in traditional medicine, it is has been used to treat respiratory infections and relieve chest congestion. Oregano essential oil contains a high content of carvacrol and thymol, two powerful compounds that are antibacterial and help loosen phlegm.[152]

Research

Antifungal: This study looked at oregano oil's antifungal properties. It was found to block the growth of Candida albicans.[153]

Antifungal–Candida albicans: Oregano, winter savory, cinnamon bark, peppermint and lemongrass were most effective against Candida albicans.[154]

Antibacterial: A group of scientists from England and India found that oregano oil was better at killing MRSA (methicillin-resistant Staphylococcus aureus) than eighteen antibiotics. The oil was effective at very low concentrations (dilution of 1 to 1000). It was potent as liquid or vapor, and still powerful used in boiling water.[155]

Antimicrobial: Black pepper, clove, geranium, nutmeg, oregano, and thyme essential oils were examined for antibacterial activity against 25 different kinds of bacteria. The oils were effective against all the tested organisms. This included bacteria that affect plants and animals and cause food poisoning and food spoilage.[156]

Safety Tips

- Do not take oregano oil by mouth.
- Do not use if pregnant or nursing.
- Use caution if you have sensitive or damaged skin.
- Do not use on children under 2 years old.
- Oregano essential oil is a powerful antimicrobial. Tisserand and Young recommend no more than 30ml (6 teaspoons) of a 1% dilution be used on the skin per day. [157]

How To Use

To use on skin: In a glass container combine carrier oil with the amount of drops needed for your desired dilution.

- To make a 1% dilution add 9 drops to 30ml (6 teaspoons) carrier oil.
- **Elderly, frail, or sensitive skin**: 0.5% dilution–Add 5 drops to 30ml (6 teaspoons) carrier oil

Ideas For Use

Diffusing: To reduce airborne-microbes, diffuse oregano oil for a few minutes in a well-ventilated room. Note the safety concern for young children and if pregnant and nursing.

Cleaning: Add a drop to your favorite cleaning products.

Laundry: To disinfect laundry, add a couple of drops to the washing machine.

References

152. Castleman, Michael. *The Healing Herbs, The Ultimate Guide to the Curative Power of Natures Medicines.* Emmaus: Rodale Press, 1991. Print page 276

153. Antifungal activities of origanum oil against Candida albicans.
Manohar V, Ingram C, Gray J, Talpur NA, Echard BW, Bagchi D, Preuss HG.
Mol Cell Biochem. 2001 Dec;228(1-2):111-7.
PMID:11855736

154. The inhibition of Candida albicans by selected essential oils and their major components.
Tampieri MP, Galuppi R, Macchioni F, Carelle MS, Falcioni L, Cioni PL, Morelli I.
Mycopathologia. 2005 Apr;159(3):339-45.
PMID:15883716

155. http://www.medicalnewstoday.com/articles/130620.php

156. Antimicrobial agents from plants: antibacterial activity of plant volatile oils.
Dorman HJ, Deans SG.
J Appl Microbiol. 2000 Feb;88(2):308-16.
PMID:10736000

157. Tisserand, Robert and Rodney Young. *Essential Oil Safety: A Guide for Health Care Professionals.* 2nd Edition. Edinburgh: Churchill Livingston Elsevier Health Sciences. 2014. Print. Page 376

Chapter 18

Patchouli
Pogostemon cablin

Botanical Family: Labiatae (mint)

Parts Used: Leaf

Country of Origin: Indonesia

Extraction Method: Steam Distillation

History and Traditional Use

Patchouli is an herb from tropical Asia that is used in fragrances, soaps and lotions.[158]

Traditionally patchouli has been used to treat colds, headaches, fever, and as an insect repellent. The essential oil is used in aromatherapy to help with depression and stress. One study found that patchouli essential oil is made up of more than 140 compounds. The study's purpose was to further understand the complexity of patchouli and its potential use in medicine.[159]

Research

Antibacterial: Previous studies have found that patchouli oil has significant antibacterial activity against methicillin-resistant Staphylococcus aureus (MRSA). Pogostone (a compound of patchouli) was evaluated and found very effective.[160]

Antiviral—Anti-influenza: In a laboratory-conducted study, patchouli alcohol (a compound found in patchouli oil) was able to inhibit influenza virus.[161]

Calming Effect: Inhalation of pepper oil, estragon oil, fennel oil or grapefruit oil had a stimulating effect on sympathetic activity (heart rate, blood pressure). Inhalation of rose oil or patchouli oil caused a 40% decrease in relative sympathetic activity (Calming effect).[162]

Insecticide and Repellent—Ants: One study tested patchouli oil against three species of ants. Patchouli was very effective at killing and repelling ants.[163]

Insecticide—Houseflies: Out of 34 tested essential oils, patchouli was the most effective against houseflies.[164]

Safety Tips
* Do not take by mouth.

How To Use
To use on skin: To make your desired dilution add drops to 30 ml carrier oil and shake or mix well. Use a glass container and an accurate measuring device, not silverware.

30 ml is the equivalent of 1 ounce or 2 tablespoons or 6 teaspoons

Elderly, Frail, Sensitive Skin	3 to 9 drops	0.5% to 1% dilution
Healthy Adults	9 to 18 drops	1% to 2% dilution
Short term on area of concern	18 to 27 drops	2% to 3% dilution

For more information on dilution please see first chapter.

Insect Repellent: Make a spray with water and a few drops of patchouli essential oil.

Diffusion: Follow the instructions that came with the diffuser. To avoid overexposure run the diffuser for only 15 to 20 minutes. Patchouli oil is often blended with other essential oils.

Direct Inhalation: Add a few drops to a handkerchief, tissue or cotton ball and inhale the aroma of the oil. If you choose to inhale the aroma directly from the bottle, hold the bottle a few inches below your nose and take a quick sniff or two. Be careful not to ingest the oil through your nose as that can be toxic.

References

158. http://www.motherearthliving.com/gardening/plant-profile/patchouli-herb-zmaz91djzgoe.aspx?Page-Id=1

159. A Comprehensive Review on the Phytochemical Constituents and Pharmacological Activities ofPogostemon cablin Benth.: An Aromatic Medicinal Plant of Industrial Importance.
Swamy MK, Sinniah UR.
Molecules. 2015 May 12;20(5):8521-8547. Review.
PMID:25985355

160. In vitro and in vivo antibacterial activity of Pogostone.
Peng F, Wan F, Xiong L, Peng C, Dai M, Chen J.
Chin Med J (Engl). 2014;127(23):4001-5.
PMID:25430439

161. Inhibitory effect and possible mechanism of action of patchouli alcohol against influenza A (H2N2) virus.
Wu H, Li B, Wang X, Jin M, Wang G.
Molecules. 2011 Aug 3;16(8):6489-501. doi: 10.3390/molecules16086489.
PMID: 21814161

162. Effects of fragrance inhalation on sympathetic activity in normal adults.
      Haze S, Sakai K, Gozu Y.
      Jpn J Pharmacol. 2002 Nov;90(3):247-53.
      PMID:12499579

163. Insecticidal and repellence activity of the essential oil of Pogostemon cablin against urban ants species.
      Albuquerque EL, Lima JK, Souza FH, Silva IM, Santos AA, Araújo AP, Blank AF, Lima RN, Alves PB, Bacci
      L.
      Acta Trop. 2013 Sep;127(3):181-6. doi: 10.1016/j.actatropica.2013.04.011. Epub 2013 Apr 30.
      PMID:23643519

164. Insecticidal properties of several essential oils on the house fly (Musca domestica L).
      Pavela R.
      Phytother Res. 2008 Feb;22(2):274-8.
      PMID:17886229

Chapter 19

Peppermint
Mentha piperita

≈≋

Botanical Family:	Lamiaceae (mint)	**Country of Origin**:	United States
Parts Used:	Leaf	**Extraction Method**:	Steam Distillation

History and Traditional Uses

Peppermint was prized by ancient Egyptians, Greeks and Romans as digestive aid. In the eighteenth century it was used for nausea, vomiting, morning sickness, respiratory infections and menstrual disorders. It reduces inflammation prevents infections and relieves pain. Inhaling peppermint's menthol vapors open nasal passageways and relieves sinus congestion.[165]

Research

Antibacterial: Peppermint and spearmint essential oils restrained the growth of antibiotic-resistant and antibiotic-sensitive strains of Helicobacter pylori and Staphylococccus aureus.[166]

Antibacterial–Respiratory Infections: Fourteen essential oils were tested against bacteria that cause respiratory infections. Thyme, cinnamon bark lemongrass, perilla, and peppermint oils were found effective and chosen for further evaluation.[167]

Antifungal–Candida albicans: Oregano, peppermint, cinnamon bark, winter savory, and lemongrass were the most active against Candida albicans.[168]

Antiviral–Herpes Simplex 1 and 2: In a laboratory-conducted study peppermint oil demonstrated a direct ability to deactivate herpes virus 1 and 2.[169]

Arthritis: Using a blend of lavender, marjoram, eucalyptus, rosemary, and peppermint oils in carrier oil significantly lowered pain and depression.[170]

Constipation: Abdominal massage with rosemary, lemon and peppermint oil helped relieve constipation.[171]

Headache: A blend of peppermint oil, eucalyptus oil and ethanol (alcohol) applied to the forehead and temple significantly reduced headache pain.[172]

Headache: The application of 10% peppermint oil in ethanol (alcohol) solution to the forehead and temple areas was as effective as taking 1000mg of acetaminophen.[173]

Insect Repellent–Paper Wasps and Yellow Jackets: A blend of clove, geranium and lemongrass oils, and also a blend of clove, geranium, lemongrass and rosemary oils totally blocked the attraction of wasps, yellow jackets and hornets.[174]

Insecticide–Houseflies: This study showed that lemongrass, peppermint and lavender essential oils have potential as an insecticide against houseflies.[175]

Insecticide–Mosquito Repellent: Dengue fever spread by the Aedes aegypti L. mosquito is a growing concern. Peppermint essential oil effectively killed the larva and repelled the mosquito that carries dengue fever.[176]

Memory–Increased Alertness: Inhalation of essential oils can produce different results. Peppermint oil was found to enhance memory and increase alertness whereas ylang-ylang essential oil was found to slow down thinking and decrease alertness, but greatly increase calmness.[177]

Mental Exhaustion: A small pilot study suggests that inhaling peppermint essential oil appears to relieve mental fatigue.[178]

Safety Tip

- Do not take by mouth.
- Tisserand and Young warn that all uses of peppermint oil should be avoided by persons who have cardiac fibrillation, or by persons with G6PD deficiency (a common genetic enzyme deficiency).
- Do not use on or close to the face of babies or children.[179]

How To Use

To use on skin: To make your desired dilution add drops to 30 ml carrier oil and shake or mix well. Use a glass container and an accurate measuring device, not silverware.

30 ml is the equivalent of 1 ounce or 2 tablespoons or 6 teaspoons

Elderly, Frail, Sensitive Skin	3 to 9 drops	0.5% to 1% dilution
Healthy Adults	9 to 18 drops	1% to 2% dilution
Short term on area of concern	18 to 27 drops	2% to 3% dilution

For more information on dilution please see first chapter.

Diffusion: Follow the instructions that came with the diffuser. To avoid overexposure, run the diffuser for only 15 to 20 minutes. **Note the safety concern for children**.

Direct Inhalation: Add a few drops to a handkerchief, tissue or cotton ball and inhale the aroma of the oil. If you choose to inhale the aroma directly from the bottle, hold the bottle a few inches below your nose and take a quick sniff or two. Be careful not to ingest the oil through your nose as that can be toxic. Note the safety concern for children.

Headache: Apply diluted oil on forehead and temples.

Insect Repellent: For immediate use make a spray with water and a few drops of peppermint oil and, if desired, other insect-repelling essential oils such as cedarwood, patchouli, geranium, lemongrass or ylang ylang.

References

165. Wurges, Jennifer; Odle, Teresa. "Peppermint." Gale Encyclopedia of Alternative Medicine. 2005.Ency-clopedia.com. 29 Jun. 2015 <http://www.encyclopedia.com>.

166. Inhibition by the essential oils of peppermint and spearmint of the growth of pathogenic bacteria.
Imai H, Osawa K, Yasuda H, Hamashima H, Arai T, Sasatsu M.
Microbios. 2001;106 Suppl 1:31-9.
PMID:11549238

167. Screening of the antibacterial effects of a variety of essential oils on respiratory tract pathogens, using a modified dilution assay method.
Inouye S, Yamaguchi H, Takizawa T.
J Infect Chemother. 2001 Dec;7(4):251-4.
PMID:11810593

168. The inhibition of Candida albicans by selected essential oils and their major components.
Tampieri MP, Galuppi R, Macchioni F, Carelle MS, Falcioni L, Cioni PL, Morelli I.
Mycopathologia. 2005 Apr;159(3):339-45.
PMID:15883716

169. Virucidal effect of peppermint oil on the enveloped viruses herpes simplex virus type 1 and type 2 in vitro.
Schuhmacher A, Reichling J, Schnitzler P.
Phytomedicine. 2003;10(6-7):504-10.
PMID:13678235

170. [The effects of aromatherapy on pain, depression, and life satisfaction of arthritis patients].
Kim MJ, Nam ES, Paik SI.
Taehan Kanho Hakhoe Chi. 2005 Feb;35(1):186-94. Korean.
PMID: 15778570

171. [Effect of aromatherapy massage for the relief of constipation in the elderly].
Kim MA, Sakong JK, Kim EJ, Kim EH, Kim EH.
Taehan Kanho Hakhoe Chi. 2005 Feb;35(1):56-64. Korean.
PMID:15778557

172. Effect of peppermint and eucalyptus oil preparations on neurophysiological and experimental algesi-metric headache parameters.
Göbel H, Schmidt G, Soyka D.
Cephalalgia. 1994 Jun;14(3):228-34; discussion 182.
PMID:7954745

173. [Effectiveness of Oleum menthae piperitae and paracetamol in therapy of headache of the tension type].
Göbel H, Fresenius J, Heinze A, Dworschak M, Soyka D.
Nervenarzt. 1996 Aug;67(8):672-81. German.
PMID:8805113

174. Essential oils and their compositions as spatial repellents for pestiferous social wasps.
Zhang QH, Schneidmiller RG, Hoover DR.
Pest Manag Sci. 2013 Apr;69(4):542-52. doi: 10.1002/ps.3411. Epub 2012 Oct 19.
PMID: 23081867

175. Efficacy of herbal essential oils as insecticides against the housefly, Musca domestica L.
Sinthusiri J, Soonwera M.
Southeast Asian J Trop Med Public Health. 2013 Mar;44(2):188-96.
PMID:23691628

176. Bioefficacy of Mentha piperita essential oil against dengue fever mosquito Aedes aegypti L.
Kumar S, Wahab N, Warikoo R.
Asian Pac J Trop Biomed. 2011 Apr;1(2):85-8. doi: 10.1016/S2221-1691(11)60001-4.
PMID: 23569733

177. Modulation of cognitive performance and mood by aromas of peppermint and ylang-ylang.
Moss M, Hewitt S, Moss L, Wesnes K.
Int J Neurosci. 2008 Jan;118(1):59-77.
PMID:18041606

178. Effect of inhaled essential oils on mental exhaustion and moderate burnout: a small pilot study.
Varney E, Buckle J.
J Altern Complement Med. 2013 Jan;19(1):69-71. doi: 10.1089/acm.2012.0089. Epub 2012 Nov 9.
PMID: 23140115

179. Tisserand, Robert and Rodney Young. *Essential Oil Safety: A Guide for Health Care Professionals.* 2nd
Edition. Edinburgh: Churchill Livingston Elsevier Health Sciences. 2014. Print. Page 387

Chapter 20

Rosemary
Rosmarinus officinalis

Botanical Family: Lamiaceae (mint)

Parts Used: Leaf

Country of Origin: Tunisia

Extraction Method: Steam Distillation

History and Traditional Uses

Rosemary is a well-know spice and medicinal herb. Traditionally it was used to enhance memory, to relieve aches and pains, and for hair growth. The German Commission E approves the use of rosemary oil to treat arthritis, muscle pain and to improve circulation.[180]

Research

Alzheimer's Disease and Dementia: Significant improvement was seen in cognitive function by using aromatherapy with rosemary and lemon essential oils in the morning, and lavender and orange essential oils in the evening.[181]

Antibacterial, Antimicrobial–Oral: Rosemary oil was found to have antimicrobial activity against microorganisms that cause dental caries (cavities in humans.[182]

Anti-inflammatory, Anti-aging: This study found that Inhalation of lavender and rosemary essential oils improved the body's free radical scavenging ability, which in turn reduced damaging oxidative stress. Oxidative stress is recognized a a harmful factor in aging and in many diseases.[183]

Arthritis: Using a blend of lavender, marjoram, eucalyptus, rosemary, and peppermint oils diluted in carrier oil significantly lowered pain and depression compared to the control group that did not use the essential oils.[184]

Constipation: Abdominal massage with rosemary, lemon and peppermint oil helps relieve constipation.[185]

Hair Growth–Alopecia Areata: Researchers had a group of men use Minoxid 2%, an over-the-counter hair loss treatment, and another group applied rosemar essential oil every day to their scalp. Both groups had significant hair growth at si months. Both groups experienced scalp itching, however the rosemary essential oil group had less scalp itching.[186]

Hair Growth–Alopecia Areata: In this study, one group massaged thyme, rosemary, lavender and cedarwood essential oils mixed with carrier oil on their scalp. The other group massaged with only carrier oil. 43% of the patients massaging the essential oils on their scalp showed improvement versus 15% improvement in the carrier-oil group.[187]

Insect Repellent–Paper Wasps and Yellow Jackets: A blend of geranium, clove and lemongrass oils, and also a blend of clove, geranium, lemongrass and rosemary oils totally blocked the attraction of wasps, yellow jackets and hornets.[188]

Memory: A 2013 study found that inhaling diffused rosemary essential oil can improve the ability to remember to do things in the future. Significant amounts of 1,8-cineole, a compound found in rosemary oil, were found in blood tests of those who inhaled the rosemary oil. This suggests that memory was improved by absorption of compounds found in rosemary essential oil.[189]

Memory: A 2003 study demonstrated that smelling rosemary essential oil significantly improved memory.[190]

Mood–Energizing: Researchers found that after inhaling rosemary oil, test subjects felt "fresher" and became more active. The results were confirmed by autonomic nervous system recordings including electroencephalography (EEG).[191]

Safety Tips

Rosemary oil can be toxic if ingested and should never be taken orally.

Do not use rosemary essential oil on or close to the face of babies or children.[192]

Do not use if pregnant or nursing.

How To Use

To use on skin: To make your desired dilution add drops to 30 ml carrier oil and shake or mix well. Use a glass container and an accurate measuring device, not silverware.

30 ml is the equivalent of 1 ounce or 2 tablespoons or 6 teaspoons

Elderly, Frail, Sensitive Skin	3 to 9 drops	0.5% to 1% dilution
Healthy Adults	9 to 18 drops	1% to 2% dilution
Short term on area of concern	18 to 27 drops	2% to 3% dilution

For more information on dilution please see first chapter.

Diffusion: Follow the instructions that came with the diffuser. To avoid overexposure run the diffuser for only 15 to 20 minutes. Note the safety concern for children and if pregnant or nursing.

Direct Inhalation: Add a few drops to a handkerchief, tissue or cotton ball and inhale the aroma of the oil. If you choose to inhale the aroma directly from the bottle, hold the bottle a few inches below your nose and take a quick sniff or two. Be careful not to ingest the oil through your nose as that can be toxic. **Note the safety concern for children and if pregnant or nursing.**

Insect Repellent: For immediate use make a spray with water and a few drops of rosemary oil and if desired, other insect-repelling essential oils such as cedarwood, patchouli, geranium, lemongrass or ylang ylang.

References

180. Rosemary | University of Maryland Medical Center http://umm.edu/health/medical/altmed/herb/rosemary#ixzz3ZmzLTBh7

181. Effect of aromatherapy on patients with Alzheimer's disease.
Jimbo D, Kimura Y, Taniguchi M, Inoue M, Urakami K.
Psychogeriatrics. 2009 Dec;9(4):173-9. doi: 10.1111/j.1479-8301.2009.00299.x.
PMID:20377818

182. Antibacterial activity of the essential oil from Rosmarinus officinalis and its major components against oral pathogens.
Bernardes WA, Lucarini R, Tozatti MG, Flauzino LG, Souza MG, Turatti IC, Andrade e Silva ML, Martins CH, da Silva Filho AA, Cunha WR.
Z Naturforsch C. 2010 Sep-Oct;65(9-10):588-93.
PMID:21138060

183. Smelling lavender and rosemary increases free radical scavenging activity and decreases cortisol level in saliva.
Atsumi T, Tonosaki K.
Psychiatry Res. 2007 Feb 28;150(1):89-96. Epub 2007 Feb 7.
PMID:17291597

184. [The effects of aromatherapy on pain, depression, and life satisfaction of arthritis patients].
Kim MJ, Nam ES, Paik SI.
Taehan Kanho Hakhoe Chi. 2005 Feb;35(1):186-94. Korean.
PMID: 15778570

185. [Effect of aromatherapy massage for the relief of constipation in the elderly].
Kim MA, Sakong JK, Kim EJ, Kim EH, Kim EH.
Taehan Kanho Hakhoe Chi. 2005 Feb;35(1):56-64. Korean.
PMID:15778557

186. Rosemary oil vs minoxidil 2% for the treatment of androgenetic alopecia: a randomized comparative trial.
Panahi Y, Taghizadeh M, Marzony ET, Sahebkar A.
Skinmed. 2015 Jan-Feb;13(1):15-21.
PMID:25842469

187. Randomized trial of aromatherapy. Successful treatment for alopecia areata.
Hay IC, Jamieson M, Ormerod AD.
Arch Dermatol. 1998 Nov;134(11):1349-52.
PMID:9828867

188. Essential oils and their compositions as spatial repellents for pestiferous social wasps.
Zhang QH, Schneidmiller RG, Hoover DR.
Pest Manag Sci. 2013 Apr;69(4):542-52. doi: 10.1002/ps.3411. Epub 2012 Oct 19.
PMID: 23081867

89. http://www.sciencedaily.com/releases/2013/04/130409091104.htm

90. Aromas of rosemary and lavender essential oils differentially affect cognition and mood in healthy adults.
Moss M. Cook J. Wesnes K. Duckett P.
Int J Neurosci. 2003 Jan;113(1):15-38.

91. Effects of inhaled rosemary oil on subjective feelings and activities of the nervous system.
Sayorwan W, Ruangrungsi N, Piriyapunyporn T, Hongratanaworakit T, Kotchabhakdi N, Siripornpan-ich V.
Sci Pharm. 2013 Jun;81(2):531-42. doi: 10.3797/scipharm.1209-05. Epub 2012 Dec 23.
PMID:23833718

92. Tisserand, Robert and Rodney Young. *Essential Oil Safety: A Guide for Health Care Professionals.* 2nd Edition. Edinburgh: Churchill Livingston Elsevier Health Sciences. 2014. Print. Page 409

Chapter 21

Sandalwood
Santalum austrocaledonicum

Botanical Family: Santalaceae

Parts Used: Wood

Country of Origin: New Caledonia

Extraction Method: Steam Distillation

History and Traditional Use

New Caledonian sandalwood essential oil is distilled from trees grown i New Caledonia in the southwest Pacific. Growing sandalwood trees provides cas income to people living in the outer islands and remote communities. Traditionall the wood is used for medicine and burnt as insect repellent. Sandalwood oil is use in cosmetics, perfumes, medicines and aromatherapy.[193]

Research

Anti-Skin Cancer: Using sandalwood oil significantly lowered the incidenc of papillomas (skin tumors) in mice, suggesting that sandalwood oil may be used a a treatment to prevent skin cancer.[194]

Herpes Simplex 1 and 2: A laboratory-conducted study found that sanda wood essential oil inhibited the replication of herpes simplex viruses 1 and 2.[195]

Sleep: Sandalwood oil is widely used in aromatherapy, as well as santalol, component of sandalwood oil that is sedating. One study done with rats as te subjects, found that santalol may be used for better sleep quality.[196]

Safety Tips

- Do not take sandalwood oil by mouth.
- Tisserand and Young recommend no more than 30ml (6 teaspoons) of a 2°
  dilution be used on the skin per day.[197]

How To Use

To use on skin, make your desired dilution by adding drops to 30 n carrier oil and shake or mix well. Use a glass container and an accurat measuring device, not silverware.

ml is the equivalent of 1 ounce or 2 tablespoons or 6 teaspoons

lerly, Frail, Sensitive Skin	3 to 9 drops	0.5% to 1% dilution
ealthy Adults	9 to 18 drops	1% to 2% dilution

For more information on dilution please see first chapter.

Diffusion: Follow the instructions that came with the diffuser. To avoid over-
osure run the diffuser for only 15 to 20 minutes.

Direct Inhalation: Add a few drops to a handkerchief, tissue or cotton ball
inhale the aroma of the oil. If you choose to inhale the aroma directly from the
tle, hold the bottle a few inches below your nose and take a quick sniff or two.
careful not to ingest the oil through your nose as that can be toxic.

Bath: Always dilute sandalwood oil if used in bath to avoid direct skin contact
h undiluted oil floating on top of the water. To use in bath add drops to a
ersing agent such as a teaspoon of whole milk or carrier oil. Then add to bath.

ferences

http://agroforestry.org/images/pdfs/Santalum-a-y-sandalwood.pdf

Chemopreventive effects of sandalwood oil on skin papillomas in mice.
Dwivedi C, Abu-Ghazaleh A.
Eur J Cancer Prev. 1997 Aug;6(4):399-401.
PMID:9370104

Antiviral activity of sandalwood oil against herpes simplex viruses-1 and -2.
Benencia F, Courrèges MC.
Phytomedicine. 1999 May;6(2):119-23.
PMID:10374251

[Effect of santalol on the sleep-wake cycle in sleep-disturbed rats].
Ohmori A, Shinomiya K, Utsu Y, Tokunaga S, Hasegawa Y, Kamei C.
Nihon Shinkei Seishin Yakurigaku Zasshi. 2007 Aug;27(4):167-71. Japanese
PMID:17879595

Tisserand, Robert and Rodney Young. *Essential Oil Safety: A Guide for Health Care Professionals*. 2nd
Edition. Edinburgh: Churchill Livingston Elsevier Health Sciences. 2014. Print. Page 419

Chapter 22

Tea Tree Oil
Melaleuca alternifolia

~~~~~

Botanical Family: Myrtaceae

Parts Used: Stems, Leaves

Country of Origin: Australia

Extraction Method: Steam Distillation

History and Traditional Use

There are over 300 known species of Melaleuca trees in Australia, bu
Melaleuca alternifolia is the only source of high quality tea tree oil. Tea tree o
distilled from the Melaleuca alternifolia tree contains over a hundred know
natural components. Terpinen-4-ol and Cineole are two of the oil's ke
components. Terpinen-4-ol is the main antimicrobial component and Cineole
a compound that makes the oil penetrating. Too much Cineole can make the o
irritating. The original high standard for tea tree oil was a minimum 35% Terpine
4-ol and a maximum 10% Cineole. Later the standard was relaxed; therefore not a
Melaleuca oils are produced according to the original high standard. Some oils ar
blends of other less effective plant species, or produced with less than 35% healir
terpinen-4-ol, or more than 10% irritating cineole.

According to legend, Aborigines living in the wetlands around Bungawalby
Creek were well aware of the medicinal qualities of their many "healing trees."
is widely understood that they treated various wounds and skin infections wit
a poultice made from crushed Melaleuca leaves and warm mud from along th
banks of the creek. They called the area where the Melaleuca trees grew an
dropped leaves into pools of waters the "healing ground."

In 1770 the "healing trees" came to be known as "tea trees" after Captain Coc
and the botanist Joseph Banks discovered they could brew a spicy and refreshir
tea with the leaves.

By the start of the second World War, tea tree oil from Melaleuca alternifol
was medically recognized world-wide for the successful treatment of ear, nos
and throat infections, tonsillitis, gingivitis, candida, thrush, fingernail and toena

fections, fungal infections, impetigo, lice, ringworm, hemorrhages and wounds. ea tree oil was also used in a variety of veterinary applications. A bottle of tea tree il was a standard Government Issue in the Australian Army and Navy first aid kits, specially for those soldiers serving in tropical countries. Traditionally tea tree oil as also been used for repelling and eradicating lice and bed bugs. Tea tree oil has een called a "first-aid kit in a bottle."

Research

Acne: 5% tea tree oil was found effective for mild to moderate acne.[198]

Allergic Skin Reactions: One study showed that tea tree oil can reduce istamine-induced skin inflammation.[199]

Antibacterial—Antiseptic/Hospital-Acquired Infections: Lemongrass was ound to be very effective against Gram-positive bacteria, while tea tree oil was ound very effective against Gram-negative bacteria. Antiseptic essential oils are nowing strong potential as affordable topical treatments to prevent multi-resistant, ospital-acquired infections.[200]

Antibacterial—Antimicrobial/Wound Care: Melaleuca alternifolia oil is ffective at treating Staphylococcus aureus, both methicillin-resistant and nethicillin-sensitive.[201]

Antibacterial—Oral: In a laboratory-conducted study Melaleuca alternifolia as found effective against a range of oral bacteria, suggesting it is useful for oral are and healthcare products.[202]

Anti-Skin Cancer: In this study cancerous skin tumors were quickly healed mice by topically applying tea tree oil combined with a chemical that increased a tree oil's skin penetration. The researchers report that clearance of tumors was result of combining tea tree oil with a product that increased deeper penetration rough the skin.[203]

Anti-Skin Cancer—Melanoma: This study reports that tea tree oil and rpinen-4-ol was able to inhibit the growth of melanoma cells.[204]

Antifungal—Athlete's Foot/Candida/Tinea/Ringworm/Dandruff: Tea tree il was effective against twenty-six strains of various dermatophyte (tinea, athlete's oot, ringworm) species, fifty-four yeasts, among them thirty-two strains of Candida bicans and other Candida species, as well as twenty-two different Malassezia rfur strains (dandruff and other skin conditions).[205]

Anti-Inflammatory, Antimicrobial, Antioxidant, Anti-Skin Cancer, eborrheic Dermatitis and Wound Healing: A review of tea tree oil's uses in ermatology found terpinen-4-ol, a natural compound found in Melaleuca alterni- lia, to have strong anti-inflammatory and antimicrobial properties. Tea tree oil an antioxidant and has anti-skin cancer properties. It is also used to treat acne, ngivitis, Seborrheic dermatitis and speeds wound healing.[206]

Antimicrobials: Vapors of tea tree oil, bergamot, lavender and eucalyptus oils hibited both bacteria and fungi.[207]

Antiviral—Anti-Influenza: Tea tree oil was found to have antiviral activity against influenza A/PR/8 virus subtype H1N1.[208]

Antiviral—Herpes Simplex 1 and 2: In a laboratory-conducted study Melaleuca oil showed high levels of antiviral activity against herpes simplex-1 and herpes simpex-2.[209]

Ear Infections: Tea tree oil has traditionally been used to treat earache and ear infections.[210]

Lice: In a laboratory-conducted study tea tree oil was able to kill 100% of lice in 30 minutes.[211]

Lice: One hundred and twenty-three children with head lice participated in this study: One group used a product made with tea tree oil and lavender oil. Another group used a "head lice suffocation product" and a third group used a product containing pyrethrins and piperonyl butoxide. The groups that used the tea tree and lavender oil product and "suffocation" product were 97.6% louse-free after the last treatment. The pyrethrins and piperonyl butoxide group were only 25% louse-free after the last treatment. [212]

Scabies: 5% TTO and its active component terpinen-4-ol were highly effective at killing scabies mites.[213]

Warts: This peer-reviewed article reports the successful treatment of warts by applying tea tree oil once-a-day for twelve days.[214]

Safety Tips

- Melaleuca oil has been safely used and held dear for many years.
- Do not take by mouth.

Although tea tree oil is often used neat (undiluted) as a first-aid treatment Tisserand and Young note that tea tree oil does have a low risk of skin sensitization. They recommend no more than 30ml (6 teaspoons) of a 15% dilution be used on the skin per day and that old or oxidized oil be avoided. Tea tree oil should be kept in a dark, airtight container in a refrigerator.[215]

How To Use

To use on skin: In a glass container combine carrier oil with the amount of drops needed for your desired dilution. 30ml equals 6 teaspoons or 2 tablespoons.
- To make a 5% dilution add 45 drops to 30ml (2 tablespoons) carrier oil.

For smaller quantities:
- To make a 5% dilution add 8 drops to 1 teaspoon carrier oil
- To make a 10% dilution add 15 drops to 1 teaspoon carrier oil
- To make a 15% dilution add 23 drops to 1 teaspoon carrier oil

Bath: Add a few diluted drops in a bath

To fight a cold and get ready for bed: add 1 cup Epsom Salts to a warm bath. Combine 3 drops tea tree oil, 3 drops eucalyptus oil and 3 drops lavender oil i

0ml carrier oil. (6 teaspoons) Massage on arms and legs. Relax in a warm bath.

Diffusion: Follow instructions that came with the diffuser. To avoid over xposure to essential oils, run the diffuser no more than 15 minutes.

Direct Inhalation: Add a few drops to a handkerchief, tissue or cotton ball nd inhale the aroma of the oil. If you choose to inhale the aroma directly from the ottle, hold the bottle a few inches below your nose and take a quick sniff or two. e careful not to ingest the oil through your nose as that can be toxic.

Earache: One drop of high quality tea tree oil (use only high quality) can be nixed with 15 to 20 drops of olive oil or other neutral oil. Insert the oil mixture irectly into the outside ear canal with a dropper. **NEVER drip pure, undiluted, il into the ear canal.**

Room Spray: Combine in a glass spray bottle or plant mister: 4 tablespoons istilled water, 2 tablespoons vodka and 20 to 30 drops of desired essential oil. nake well before each use.

Laundry: Add a few drops to laundry or rinse water when cleaning.

eferences

8. The efficacy of 5% topical tea tree oil gel in mild to moderate acne vulgaris: a randomized, dou-ble-blind placebo-controlled study.
Enshaieh S, Jooya A, Siadat AH, Iraji F.
Indian J Dermatol Venereol Leprol. 2007 Jan-Feb;73(1):22-5.

9. Tea tree oil reduces histamine-induced skin inflammation.
Koh KJ, Pearce AL, Marshman G, Finlay-Jones JJ, Hart PH.
Br J Dermatol. 2002 Dec;147(6):1212-7.
PMID:12452873

00. The ongoing battle against multi-resistant strains: in-vitro inhibition of hospital-acquired MRSA, VRE, Pseudomonas, ESBL E. coli and Klebsiella species in the presence of plant-derived antiseptic oils.
Warnke PH, Lott AJ, Sherry E, Wiltfang J, Podschun R.
J Craniomaxillofac Surg. 2013 Jun;41(4):321-6. doi: 10.1016/j.jcms.2012.10.012. Epub 2012 Nov 29.
PMID:23199627

01. Staphylococcus aureus and wounds: a review of tea tree oil as a promising antimicrobial.
Halcón L, Milkus K.
Am J Infect Control. 2004 Nov;32(7):402-8. Review.
PMID:15525915

02. Susceptibility of oral bacteria to Melaleuca alternifolia (tea tree) oil in vitro.
Hammer KA, Dry L, Johnson M, Michalak EM, Carson CF, Riley TV.
Oral Microbiol Immunol. 2003 Dec;18(6):389-92.
PMID:14622345

03. Topically applied Melaleuca alternifolia (tea tree) oil causes direct anti-cancer cytotoxicity in subcuta-neous tumour bearing mice.
Ireland DJ, Greay SJ, Hooper CM, Kissick HT, Filion P, Riley TV, Beilharz MW.
J Dermatol Sci. 2012 Aug;67(2):120-9. doi: 10.1016/j.jdermsci.2012.05.005. Epub 2012 May 27.
PMID:22727730

04. Tea tree oil might combat melanoma.
Bozzuto G, Colone M, Toccacieli L, Stringaro A, Molinari A.
Planta Med. 2011 Jan;77(1):54-6. doi: 10.1055/s-0030-1250055. Epub 2010 Jun 17.
PMID:20560116

205. Antifungal activity of essential oil of Melaleuca alternifolia (tea tree oil) against pathogenic fungi in vitro.
Nenoff P, Haustein UF, Brandt W.
Skin Pharmacol. 1996;9(6):388-94.
PMID:9055360

206. A review of applications of tea tree oil in dermatology.
Pazyar N, Yaghoobi R, Bagherani N, Kazerouni A.
Int J Dermatol. 2013 Jul;52(7):784-90. doi: 10.1111/j.1365-4632.2012.05654.x. Epub 2012 Sep 24.
Review.
PMID: 22998411

207. Vapour phase: a potential future use for essential oils as antimicrobials?
Laird K, Phillips C.
Lett Appl Microbiol. 2012 Mar;54(3):169-74. doi: 10.1111/j.1472-765X.2011.03190.x. Epub 2012 Jan 6.
PMID:22133088

208. In vitro antiviral activity of Melaleuca alternifolia essential oil.
Garozzo A, Timpanaro R, Bisignano B, Furneri PM, Bisignano G, Castro A.
Lett Appl Microbiol. 2009 Dec;49(6):806-8. doi: 10.1111/j.1472-765X.2009.02740.x. Epub 2009 Sep 18.
PMID: 19843207

209. Antiviral activity of Australian tea tree oil and eucalyptus oil against herpes simplex virus in cell culture.
Schnitzler P, Schön K, Reichling J.
Pharmazie. 2001 Apr;56(4):343-7.
PMID:11338678

210. http://www.livestrong.com/article/474412-ear-aches-tea-tree-oil/

211. Activity of tea tree oil and nerolidol alone or in combination against Pediculus capitis (head lice) and its eggs.
Di Campli E, Di Bartolomeo S, Delli Pizzi P, Di Giulio M, Grande R, Nostro A, Cellini L.
Parasitol Res. 2012 Nov;111(5):1985-92. doi: 10.1007/s00436-012-3045-0. Epub 2012 Jul 31.
PMID:22847279

212. A randomised, assessor blind, parallel group comparative efficacy trial of three products for the treatment of head lice in children--melaleuca oil and lavender oil, pyrethrins and piperonyl butoxide, and "suffocation" product.
Barker SC, Altman PM.
BMC Dermatol. 2010 Aug 20;10:6. doi: 10.1186/1471-5945-10-6.
PMID: 20727129

213. Acaricidal activity of Melaleuca alternifolia (tea tree) oil: in vitro sensitivity of sarcoptes scabiei var hominis to terpinen-4-ol.
Walton SF, McKinnon M, Pizzutto S, Dougall A, Williams E, Currie BJ.
Arch Dermatol. 2004 May;140(5):563-6.
PMID:15148100

214. Successful topical treatment of hand warts in a paediatric patient with tea tree oil (Melaleuca alternifolia).
Millar BC, Moore JE.
Complement Ther Clin Pract. 2008 Nov;14(4):225-7. doi: 10.1016/j.ctcp.2008.05.003. Epub 2008 Jul 11.
PMID:18940708

215. Tisserand, Robert and Rodney Young. *Essential Oil Safety: A Guide for Health Care Professionals*. 2nd Edition. Edinburgh: Churchill Livingston Elsevier Health Sciences. 2014. Print. Page 441

216. http://www.epsomsaltcouncil.org/news/articles/doctors_say_treat_colds_flu_with_epsom_salt.php

Chapter 23

Wintergreen

Gaultheria procumbens

Botanical Family:	Ericaceae	**Country of Origin**:	United States
Parts Used:	Leaf	**Extraction Method**:	Steam Distillation

History and Traditional Use

Wintergreen is extracted from a low growing shiny-leaf shrub that is not related to mint. It is an attractive ground cover that grows in the eastern part of the United States and Canada. North American Indians used the wintergreen leaves to treat achy muscles and joints. The leaves were also used for headaches and inflammation. Wintergreen contains methyl salicylate which is related to aspirin (acetylsalicylic acid). Today it is used in topical pain killers. Most wintergreen flavoring used today comes from synthetic methyl salicylate.[217]

Research

Acute Pain: This review concludes that using topical salicylates for acute pain was significantly better than using a placebo.[218]

Safety Tips

Do not take by mouth; for external use only.

Do not use if pregnant or nursing.

Do not use on children. 4-10 ml of wintergreen by mouth can be deadly.

Do not use if you have a salicylate or aspirin allergy.

Do not use if you are taking Warfarin (Coumadin)

Do not use large amounts of wintergreen oil if you are also taking aspirin.

Do not use on diseased, damaged or broken skin.

Always use diluted with carrier oil. [219]

Tisserand and Young recommend no more than 30ml (6 teaspoons) of a 2.4% dilution be used on the skin per day.[220]

How To Use

To use on skin: In a glass container combine carrier oil with the amount of drops needed for your desired dilution.

- To make a 2.4% dilution add 22 drops to 30ml (6 teaspoons) carrier oil. Massage on areas of concern.

References

217. http://cms.herbalgram.org/healthyingredients/Wintergreen.html?ts=1433882425&signature=49aa6bd-f8bf5d46a9a6fa72ed1010e38

218. Systematic review of efficacy of topical rubefacients containing salicylates for the treatment of acute and chronic pain.
Mason L, Moore RA, Edwards JE, McQuay HJ, Derry S, Wiffen PJ.
BMJ. 2004 Apr 24;328(7446):995. Epub 2004 Mar 19. Review.
PMID:15033879

219. http://www.webmd.com/vitamins-supplements/ingredientmono-783-wintergreen.aspx?activeingredientid=783&activeingredientname=wintergreen

220. Tisserand, Robert and Rodney Young. *Essential Oil Safety: A Guide for Health Care Professionals.* 2nd Edition. Edinburgh: Churchill Livingston Elsevier Health Sciences. 2014. Print. Page 469

Ylang Ylang
Cananga odorata

Botanical Family:	Annonaceae (Custard Apple)	**Country of Origin:**	Nosy Be, Madagascar
Parts Used:	Flower	**Extraction Method:**	Steam Distillation

History and Traditional Use

Nosy Be is an island off the northwest coast of Madagascar where Cananga odorata trees, also known as perfume trees, are grown. Ylang ylang essential oil is extracted from the sweet-scented exotic flowers.[221]

Research

Blood Pressure: One study found that healthy men who inhaled ylang ylang had a reduction in heart rate and blood pressure. A sedative effect was also seen.[222]

Blood Pressure—Stress: Persons with essential hypertension who inhaled a combination of lavender, ylang-ylang and bergamot essential oils once daily were able to reduce psychological stress as well as blood pressure.[223]

Blood Pressure: In one study prehypertensive and hypertensive subjects inhaled a blend of lavender, ylang ylang, marjoram and neroli. Daytime blood pressure readings were significantly reduced and subjects were more relaxed than the placebo and control groups.[224]

Blood Pressure—Calm and Alert: This study found that inhalation of ylang-ylang essential oil significantly reduced blood pressure and heart rate. The subjects reported that they felt more alert yet calm. Researchers used the term "harmonization" instead of sedation or relaxation to describe the results achieved by inhalation of ylang ylang oil.[225]

Blood Pressure—Depression and Stress: Ylang Ylang applied to the skin significantly reduced blood pressure and increased skin temperature. It was relaxing and calming. This study provides evidence for using ylang ylang for depression and stress.[226]

Mood—Calmness: Inhalation of essential oils can produce different result Peppermint oil was found to enhance memory and increase alertness, where: ylang-ylang essential oil was found to slow down thinking and decrease alertne but greatly increase calmness.[227]

Insect Repellent: Ylang ylang and lemongrass essential oil were examine as repellents against two mosquito vectors (Aedes aegypti L. and Culex quinc uefasciatus). The research concluded that both oils can be used as safe mosqui repellents.[228]

Safety Tips

- Do not take ylang ylang oil by mouth.
- Use caution with sensitive or damaged skin.
- Do not use with children under two years of age.
- If used too frequently on skin, without enough dilution or on skin that damaged, ylang ylang can trigger the immune system to identify the oil harmful and cause an allergy-like inflammatory reaction. This reaction is mo common in persons who tend to have allergies.
- Tisserand and Young recommend no more than 30ml (6 teaspoons) of 0.8% dilution be used on the skin per day.[229]

How To Use

To use on skin: In a glass container combine carrier oil with the amount drops needed for your desired dilution. 30ml equals 6 teaspoons or 2 tablespoor

- To make a 0.8% dilution add 7 drops to 30ml (6 teaspoons) carrier oil.
- To make a smaller amount of a 0.8% dilution add 1 drop to 1 teaspoon (5n carrier oil.

Diffusion: Follow the instructions that came with the diffuser. To avoid ove exposure run the diffuser for only 15 to 20 minutes. Do not use with childre under the age of two.

Direct Inhalation: Add a few drops to a handkerchief, tissue or cotton b. and inhale the aroma of the oil. If you choose to inhale the aroma directly from tl bottle, hold the bottle a few inches below your nose and take a quick sniff or tw Be careful not to ingest the oil through your nose as that can be toxic.

Insect Repellent: For immediate use make a spray with water and a few dro| of ylang ylang and if desired other insect-repelling essential oils such as cedarwoc peppermint, patchouli, geranium or lemongrass.

Room Spray: Combine in a glass spray bottle or plant mister: 4 tablespoo distilled water, 2 tablespoons vodka and 20 to 30 drops of desired essential c Shake well before each use.

References

221. ylang-ylang. (2015). In *Encyclopædia Britannica*. Retrieved fromhttp://www.britannica.com/EBchecked/topic/653363/ylang-ylang

222. Effects of Ylang-Ylang aroma on blood pressure and heart rate in healthy men.
Jung DJ, Cha JY, Kim SE, Ko IG, Jee YS.
J Exerc Rehabil. 2013 Apr;9(2):250-5. doi: 10.12965/jer.130007. Epub 2013 Apr 25. PMID: 24278868

223. [The effects of the inhalation method using essential oils on blood pressure and stress responses of clients with essential hypertension].
Hwang JH.
Taehan Kanho Hakhoe Chi. 2006 Dec;36(7):1123-34. Korean.

224. Essential oil inhalation on blood pressure and salivary cortisol levels in prehypertensive and hypertensive subjects.
Kim IH, Kim C, Seong K, Hur MH, Lim HM, Lee MS.

225. Evaluation of the harmonizing effect of ylang-ylang oil on humans after inhalation.
Hongratanaworakit T, Buchbauer G.
Planta Med. 2004 Jul;70(7):632-6.
PMID: 15303255

226. Relaxing effect of ylang ylang oil on humans after transdermal absorption.
Hongratanaworakit T, Buchbauer G.
Phytother Res. 2006 Sep;20(9):758-63.
PMID: 16807875

227. Modulation of cognitive performance and mood by aromas of peppermint and ylang-ylang.
Moss M, Hewitt S, Moss L, Wesnes K.
Int J Neurosci. 2008 Jan;118(1):59-77.
PMID: 18041606

228. Efficacy of Thai herbal essential oils as green repellent against mosquito vectors.
Soonwera M, Phasomkusolsil S.
Acta Trop. 2015 Feb;142:127-30. doi: 10.1016/j.actatropica.2014.11.010. Epub 2014 Nov 28.
PMID:25438256

229. Tisserand, Robert and Rodney Young. *Essential Oil Safety: A Guide for Health Care Professionals*. 2nd Edition. Edinburgh: Churchill Livingston Elsevier Health Sciences. 2014. Print. Page 478

Problems Index

A

Acne
Orange 50
Tea Tree Oil 69

Allergic skin reactions
Tea Tree Oil 69

Alzheimer's disease
Lavender 34
Lemon 40
Orange 50
Rosemary 62

Analgesic (to relieve pain)
Eucalyptus 20
Lavender 34
Marjoram 46
Orange 51
Peppermint 58
Rosemary 62
Wintergreen 73

Anesthetic
Clove 17
Myrrh 48

Anti-aging - reduces oxidative stress
Lavender 34
Rosemary 62

Anti-aging - skin treatment
Grapefruit 29
Lemon 40
Myrrh 48

Antibacterial - air disinfectant
Bergamot 8
Eucalyptus 20
Geranium 26
Lavender 34

Lemongrass 43
Orange 51
Oregano 53
Tea Tree Oil 71

Antibacterial - antimicrobial
Bergamot 8
Cinnamon Bark 15
Clove 17
Eucalyptus 20
Geranium 26
Lavender 34
Lemon 40
Lemongrass 43
Myrrh 48
Orange 50
Oregano 53
Patchouli 55
Peppermint 58
Rosemary 62
Tea Tree Oil 69

Antibacterial - hospital acquired infections
Cinnamon Bark 14
Lemongrass 43
Tea Tree Oil 69

Antibacterial - oral
Clove 17
Rosemary 62
Tea Tree Oil 69

Antibacterial - respiratory infections
Cinnamon Bark 14
Eucalyptus 20
Lemongrass 43
Peppermint 58
Tea Tree Oil 69

Antifungal
Cedarwood 11
Cinnamon Bark 14
Eucalyptus 20
Frankincense 24
Geranium 27
Lavender 34
Lemon 40
Lemongrass 43
Oregano 53
Peppermint 58
Tea Tree Oil 69

Anti-inflammatory
Cedarwood 11
Eucalyptus 20
Lavender 34
Orange 50
Peppermint 58
Rosemary 62
Tea Tree Oil 69

Antiseptic
Cedarwood 11
Clove 17
Lavender 34
Myrrh 48
Tea Tree Oil 69

Anti-skin cancer
Sandalwood 66
Tea Tree Oil 69

Antitumor
Cinnamon Bark 15
Myrrh 48

Antiviral - anti-influenza
Patchouli 55
Tea Tree Oil 69

Mental fatigue
  Peppermint 59
Migraine headache
  Lavender 35
Mood - relaxing,
  calming
  Cedarwood 11
  Jasmine 32
  Lavender 34
  Patchouli 55
  Ylang Ylang 75
Mood - stimulating
  Grapefruit 29
  Jasmine 32
  Peppermint 59
  Rosemary 63
Morning sickness -
  pregnancy
  Lemon 41
  Peppermint 58

P
Pain relief,
  See **Analgesic (to**
  relieve pain)
Periodontal disease,
  See **Tooth decay**

Premenstrual
  syndrome
  Lavender 36

R
Respiratory Infection,
  See **Antibacterial**
  - respiratory
  infections
Ringworm
  Bergamot 8
  Tea Tree Oil 68, 69

S
Scabies
  Clove 18
  Tea Tree Oil 70
Sinusitis
  Eucalyptus 20
  Lavender 34
  Peppermint 58
Sleep
  Lavender 35
  Marjoram 46
  Sandalwood 66

Stress
  Bergamot 8
  Lavender 34, 35
  Orange 50
  Patchouli 55
  Ylang Ylang 75

T
Tinea
  Tea Tree Oil 69
Tooth decay
  Clove 18
  Myrrh 48
  Rosemary 62
  Tea Tree Oil 69

W
Warts
  Tea Tree Oil 70
Weight loss
  Grapefruit 29, 30
  Lemon 41
Wound healing -
  antibacterial
  Cedarwood 11
  Geranium 26
  Lavender 34
  Tea Tree Oil 68, 69

Order Information
RM Barry Publications, LLC
1 (888) 209-0510
www.rmbarry.com

Quantity Pricing
(US Dollars)

Quantity	Price Each
1–4	$5.95
5–9	$5.25
10–24	$4.60
25–49	$3.95
50+	$3.25